Pharmacology

Editor

REBECCA MAXSON

PHYSICIAN ASSISTANT CLINICS

www.physicianassistant.theclinics.com

Consulting Editors
KIM ZUBER
JANE S. DAVIS

April 2023 • Volume 8 • Number 2

ELSEVIER

1600 John F. Kennedy Boulevard • Suite 1800 • Philadelphia, Pennsylvania, 19103-2899

http://www.theclinics.com

PHYSICIAN ASSISTANT CLINICS Volume 8, Number 2
April 2023 ISSN 2405-7991, ISBN-13: 978-0-323-96077-9

Editor: Taylor Hayes
Developmental Editor: Axell Ivan Jade Purificacion

Physician Assistant Clinics (ISSN: 2405–7991) is published quarterly by Elsevier Inc., 360 Park Avenue South, New York, NY 10010-1710. Months of issue are January, April, July, and October. Periodicals postage paid at New York, NY and additional mailing offices. Subscription prices are $150.00 per year (US individuals), $305.00 (US institutions), $100.00 (US students), $150.00 (Canadian individuals), $320.00 (Canadian institutions), $100.00 (Canadian students), $150.00 (international individuals), $320.00 (international institutions), and $100.00 (international students). Foreign air speed delivery is included in all *Clinics* subscription prices. All prices are subject to change without notice. POSTMASTER: Send address changes to *Physician Assistant Clinics*, Elsevier Periodicals Customer Service, 11830 Westline Industrial Drive, St. Louis, MO 63146. Customer Service Health Sciences Division, Subscription Customer Service, 3251 Riverport Lane, Maryland Heights, MO 63043. **Customer Service: 1-800-654-2452 (U.S. and Canada); 314-447-8871 (outside U.S. and Canada). Fax: 314-447-8029. E-mail: journalscustomerservice-usa@elsevier.com (for print support); journalsonlinesupport-usa@elsevier.com (for online support).**

Reprints. For copies of 100 or more, of articles in this publication, please contact the Commercial Reprints Department, Elsevier Inc., 360 Park Avenue South, New York, NY 10010-1710. Tel. 212-633-3874; Fax: 212-633-3820; E-mail: reprints@elsevier.com.

Physician Assistant Clinics is covered in *EMBASE/Excerpta Medica and ESCI*.

PROGRAM OBJECTIVE

The goal of the *Physician Assistant Clinics* is to keep practicing physician assistants up to date with current clinical practice by providing timely articles reviewing the state of the art in patient care.

TARGET AUDIENCE

Physician Assistants and other healthcare professionals

LEARNING OBJECTIVES

Upon completion of this activity, participants will be able to:

1. Review history of pharmacotherapeutics and evolution to patents.
2. Discuss best practices in prescribing medications in adults and explain how insurance can impact the medication pipeline.
3. Recognize common treatments for cardiac, gut, and kidney health.

ACCREDITATION

The Elsevier Office of Continuing Medical Education (EOCME) is accredited by the Accreditation Council for Continuing Medical Education (ACCME) to provide continuing medical education for physicians.

The EOCME designates this journal-based CME activity for a maximum of 13 *AMA PRA Category 1 Credit*(s)™. Physicians should claim only the credit commensurate with the extent of their participation in the activity.

All other health care professionals requesting continuing education credit for this enduring material will be issued a certificate of participation.

DISCLOSURE OF CONFLICTS OF INTEREST

The EOCME assesses conflict of interest with its instructors, faculty, planners, and other individuals who are in a position to control the content of CME activities. All relevant conflicts of interest that are identified are thoroughly vetted by EOCME for fair balance, scientific objectivity, and patient care recommendations. EOCME is committed to providing its learners with CME activities that promote improvements or quality in healthcare and not a specific proprietary business or a commercial interest.

The planning committee, staff, authors, and editors listed below have identified no financial relationships or relationships to products or devices they or their spouse/life partner have with commercial interest related to the content of this CME activity:

Rebecca Boyle, MSPA, PA-C; Jane S. Davis, CRNP, DNP; Julie E. Farrar, PharmD, CCCP; Kenda E. Germain, PharmD, BCPS; Shelton K. Givens; Sarah S. Harlan, PharmD, BCCCP; Amber M. Hutchison, PharmD, BCPS, BCGP; Rebecca Johnson, PA-C; Lynette Jones, MSN, RN-BC; Mattie C. Kilpatrick; Pradeep Kuttysankaran; Jessica M. Lungen; Rebecca Maxson, PharmD; Lena McDowell, PharmD; Alyssa J. Osmonson, PharmD; Valerie Prince, PharmD, BCPS, FAPhA; Lauren Remer, MSPA, PA-S; Lavinia Salama, PharmD; Jeanna Sewell, PharmD; Steven Sica, PharmD; Sean Smithgall, PharmD, BCACP; Jessica Starr, PharmD, BCPS; Victoria Trott, PA-C, MMS; Kara A. Valentine, MMS, PA-C; Courtney S. Watts Alexander, PharmD, BCPS, BCOP; Mafe Zmajevac, PharmD

The planning committee, staff, authors, and editors listed below have identified financial relationships or relationships to products or devices they or their spouse/life partner have with commercial interest related to the content of this CME activity:

Katie E. Cardone, PharmD, BCACP, FNKF, FASN, FCCP: Advisor: AstraZeneca, Otsuka, Vifor

Emily R. Hajjar, PharmD, MS, BCPS, BCACP, BCGP: Researcher: Ethos

Brooke K. Worster, MS, FACP: Researcher: Ethos; Advisor: PAX Labs, Inc.

UNAPPROVED/OFF-LABEL USE DISCLOSURE

The EOCME requires CME faculty to disclose to the participants:

1. When products or procedures being discussed are off-label, unlabelled, experimental, and/or investigational (not US Food and Drug Administration [FDA] approved); and
2. Any limitations on the information presented, such as data that are preliminary or that represent ongoing research, interim analyses, and/or unsupported opinions. Faculty may discuss information about pharmaceutical agents that is outside of FDA-approved labelling. This information is intended solely for CME and is not intended to promote off-label use of these medications. If you have any questions, contact the medical affairs department of the manufacturer for the most recent prescribing information.

TO ENROLL

The CME program is available to all *Physician Assistant Clinics* subscribers at no additional fee. To subscribe to the *Physician Assistant Clinics*, call customer service at 1-800-654-2452 or sign up online at www.physicianassistant.theclinics.com/.

METHOD OF PARTICIPATION

In order to claim credit, participants must complete the following:

1. Complete enrolment as indicated above
2. Read the activity
3. Complete the CME Test and Evaluation. Participants must achieve a score of 70% on the test. All CME Tests and Evaluations must be completed online

CME INQUIRIES/SPECIAL NEEDS

For all CME inquiries or special needs, please contact elsevierCME@elsevier.com.

Contributors

CONSULTING EDITORS

KIM ZUBER, PAC, MS
Executive Director, American Academy of Nephrology PAs, St Petersburg, Florida

JANE S. DAVIS, CRNP, DNP
Division of Nephrology, University of Alabama at Birmingham, Birmingham, Alabama

EDITOR

REBECCA MAXSON, PharmD, BCPS
Associate Clinical Professor, Department of Pharmacy Practice, Auburn University Harrison College of Pharmacy, Birmingham, Alabama

AUTHORS

REBECCA BOYLE, MSPA, PA-C
Inpatient Medicine, Stanford Healthcare, Stanford, California

KATIE E. CARDONE, PharmD, BCACP, FNKF, FASN, FCCP
Associate Professor, Albany College of Pharmacy and Health Sciences, Albany, New York

JANE S. DAVIS, CRNP, DNP
Division of Nephrology, The University of Alabama at Birmingham, Birmingham, Alabama

JULIE E. FARRAR, PharmD, BCCCP
Assistant Professor, University of Tennessee College of Pharmacy, Memphis, Tennessee

KENDA E. GERMAIN, PharmD, BCPS
Clinical Pharmacy Specialist, Department of Pharmacy, Princeton Baptist Medical Center, Birmingham, Alabama

SHELTON K. GIVENS, PharmD
Candidate 2023, Auburn University Harrison College of Pharmacy, Auburn University, Alabama

EMILY R. HAJJAR, PharmD, MS, BCPS, BCACP, BCGP
Professor, Jefferson College of Pharmacy, Thomas Jefferson University, Philadelphia, Pennsylvania

SARAH S. HARLAN, PharmD, BCCCP
Clinical Pharmacy Specialist, Baptist Memorial Hospital–Memphis, Memphis, Tennessee

AMBER M. HUTCHISON, PharmD, BCPS, BCGP
Associate Clinical Professor, Auburn University, Harrison College of Pharmacy, Auburn, Alabama

REBECCA JOHNSON, PA-C
Clinician, Mercy Medical Clinic, Auburn, Alabama

MATTIE C. KILPATRICK, PharmD
Candidate 2023, Auburn University Harrison College of Pharmacy, Auburn University, Alabama

JESSICA M. LUNGEN, PharmD Candidate
Candidate, Jefferson College of Pharmacy, Thomas Jefferson University, Philadelphia, Pennsylvania

LENA McDOWELL, PharmD
Assistant Clinical Professor, Auburn University Harrison College of Pharmacy, Auburn University, Alabama

ALYSSA J. OSMONSON, PharmD, BCPS
Clinical Pharmacy Specialist, Department of Pharmacy, Princeton Baptist Medical Center, Birmingham, Alabama

VALERIE PRINCE, PharmD, BCPS, FAPhA
Professor of Pharmacy Practice, Samford University McWhorter School of Pharmacy, Clinical Specialist, St Vincent's East Family Medicine Residency Program, Christ Health Center, Odenville, Alabama

LAUREN REMER, MSPA, PA-S
Inpatient Medicine, Stanford Health Care - ValleyCare, Pleasanton, California

LAVINIA SALAMA, PharmD
Clinical Assistant Professor of Pharmacy Practice, University of Wyoming School of Pharmacy, Cheyenne, Wyoming

JEANNA SEWELL, PharmD
Clinical Assistant Professor, Director of Interprofessional Education, Department of Pharmacy Practice, Auburn University Harrison School of Pharmacy, Auburn, Alabama

STEVEN SICA, PharmD
Ambulatory Care Clinical Pharmacist, Yale New Haven Health, New Haven, Connecticut

SEAN SMITHGALL, PharmD, BCACP
Associate Clinical Professor, Auburn University Harrison College of Pharmacy, Mobile, Alabama

JESSICA STARR, PharmD, BCPS
Associate Clinical Professor, Auburn University Harrison School of Pharmacy, Auburn, Alabama

VICTORIA TROTT, PA-C, MMS
Physician Assistant, Annapolis Neurology Associates, Annapolis, Maryland

KARA A. VALENTINE, MMS, PA-C
Assistant Professor, Physician Assistant Program, West Palm Beach, Florida

COURTNEY S. WATTS ALEXANDER, PharmD, BCPS, BCOP
Assistant Professor, Auburn University Harrison College of Pharmacy, Auburn University, Alabama

BROOKE K. WORSTER, MD, FACP
Associate Professor, Division Director, Supportive Oncology, Program Director, Medical Cannabis Science and Business, Sidney Kimmel Medical College, Thomas Jefferson University, Philadelphia, Pennsylvania

MAFE ZMAJEVAC, PharmD
Ambulatory Care Pharmacist, Auburn University Pharmaceutical Care Center, Auburn University, Alabama

Contents

Foreword: The Essential Pharmacist **xv**

Kim Zuber and Jane S. Davis

Preface: Medications: Do Good and Avoid Bad **xvii**

Rebecca Maxson

Pharmacy Through the Ages: From Potions to Patents **237**

Jane S. Davis

Evidence from prehistoric times show the use of plants and herbs to treat human and animal ills. Today's pharmacist is highly trained and educated in the chemistry, physiology, and the dispensing of substances used to treat conditions ranging from insect bites to the most complex conditions. It has been an interesting journey from the village herbalist to today's practitioner.

Medications for When the Heart Fails **243**

Kenda E. Germain and Alyssa J. Osmonson

Heart failure is a chronic disease that carries a significant public health burden. Optimizing medication regimens in patients with heart failure with reduced ejection fraction through the use of guideline-directed medical therapy leads to positive benefits on morbidity and mortality and is paramount to optimizing outcomes. In patients with heart failure with reduced ejection fraction, the use of an angiotensin II receptor blocker with neprilysin inhibitor (or angiotensin-converting enzyme inhibitor/angiotensin receptor blocker) in addition to an evidenced-based beta-blocker, aldosterone antagonist, and sodium–glucose cotransporter 2 inhibitor is the mainstay of therapy.

Medications When the Brain Is Hurt **259**

Jessica Starr and Victoria Trott

Ischemic stroke presents as an acute onset of focal neurologic deficit. Risk factors include hypertension, diabetes, dyslipidemia, atrial fibrillation, and cigarette smoking. tPA and aspirin are the two primary agents recommended for acute treatment. recombinant tissue plasminogen activator is recommended within 4.5 hours of symptom onset because of its ability to achieve early reperfusion. Aspirin, clopidogrel, and extended-release dipyridamole plus aspirin are antiplatelet options for secondary prevention. Intracerebral hemorrhage is the second most common subtype of stroke. Basic life support is the initial step, followed by medications to control seizures, blood pressure, intracranial pressure, and bleeding.

Managing Diabetes 269

Jeanna Sewell and Rebecca Johnson

Type 2 diabetes is a complex condition with a large public health impact. The management of this condition can be intimidating due to changes in guidelines and drug therapy options. There are several newer drug therapies on the market for treatment of type 2 diabetes, many of which have a positive impact on other comorbid conditions as well. Guidance is available for when to use each therapy for the best clinical outcomes for patients.

Therapeutic Benefits of Medical Cannabis 281

Emily R. Hajjar, Jessica M. Lungen, and Brooke K. Worster

Cannabis has been used medicinally and recreationally for centuries. More recently, states have begun to allow the legal use of medical marijuana or cannabis. The two major cannabinoids are tetrahydrocannabinol (THC) and cannabidiol (CBD). Evidence suggests that the use of cannabis may be helpful in treating certain types of pain, insomnia, anxiety, nausea, and anorexia among other conditions.

Pharmacotherapeutic Management of Hypertensive Crisis 293

Sarah S. Harlan and Julie E. Farrar

Hypertensive crisis is an acute blood pressure increase to greater than 180/120 mm Hg and is broken down into 2 subcategories. End-organ damage manifests in hypertensive emergency (HTN-E) as the result of the acute elevation in blood pressure, and hypertensive urgency (HTN-U) is the absence of end-organ damage despite blood pressures greater than 180/120 mm Hg. Intravenous antihypertensive agents are used in HTN-E to lower blood pressure and prevent further organ damage. Oral antihypertensives may decrease blood pressure more slowly in HTN-U, which typically stems from lack of compliance with outpatient medication regimens for known hypertension.

Best Practices in Medical Management of Chronic Hypertension 305

Rebecca Boyle and Lauren Remer

Firmly establishing the diagnosis of hypertension and exclusion of potential causes of secondary hypertension is essential in ensuring the appropriate initial prescription of medication to lower blood pressure. Identifying patient populations with compelling indications for specific classes of antihypertensives can help prioritize medical therapies with proven clinical benefit. Finally, understanding the basic physiologic mechanisms of first- and second-line agents can facilitate the selection of medications with the greatest risk/benefit ratio.

Prescribing Across Adulthood 319

Kara A. Valentine and Amber M. Hutchison

Across adulthood, the need and use of prescribed medications increases, especially in the older patient. Medical providers should consider several factors and use a patient-centered approach. This process should be guided by the principles of appropriate prescribing and recommended

treat, or even prevent the incidence of specific diseases. Pharmacogenomics, an essential aspect of precision medicine, uses information gained from genetic testing to analyze drug-gene interactions and can improve patient outcomes by optimizing efficacy and mitigating adverse drug effects.

Explaining Insurance and the Medication Pipeline **391**

Lena McDowell and Mafe Zmajevac

Medications are essential components to patients' health-care regimens, and prescription drug costs account for approximately 9% of total health-care costs in the United States. This article provides information regarding the new drug development and approval process, health and prescription drug insurance, and how health-care providers can address social determinants of health contributing to lack of medication access and assist patients in receiving their medications.

PHYSICIAN ASSISTANT CLINICS

FORTHCOMING ISSUES

July 2023
Emerging and Re-Emerging Infectious Diseases
Gerald Kayingo, *Editor*

October 2023
Allergy, Asthma, and Immunology
Gabriel Ortiz, *Editor*

January 2024
Medicine Outside Four Walls
J. Randy Howell, *Editor*

RECENT ISSUES

January 2023
Emergency Medicine
Dan Michael Tzizik, *Editor*

October 2022
Nutrition in Patient Care
Corri Wolf, *Editor*

July 2022
Obstetrics and Gynecology
Elyse Watkins, *Editor*

SERIES OF RELATED INTEREST

Primary Care: Clinics in Office Practice
https://www.primarycare.theclinics.com/

Foreword
The Essential Pharmacist

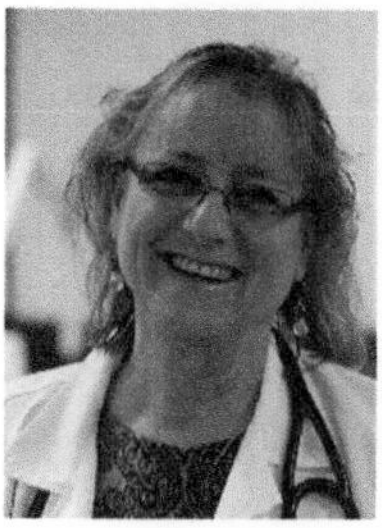
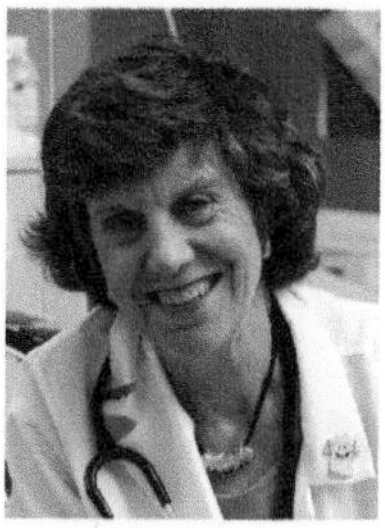

Kim Zuber, PAC, MS Jane S. Davis, CRNP, DNP
Consulting Editors

Medicine often claims to be a team effort. Yet, at times, the players have found themselves in an adversarial atmosphere instead. Over the centuries, the practice of medicine and the dispensing of medications have been intertwined and interdependent. However, despite the close relationship, there have been periods when they were more competitive than cooperative. Despite any differences, they have always been inseparable.

For the first time in the history of *Physician Assistant Clinics*, we have asked PharmDs to take an issue and teach us what they know (and they know a lot!). Many of us were lucky enough to have a PharmD on our training rotations in PA school; while others were not as fortunate. However, once we leave the university setting, a pharmacist is often not readily available to assist in patient management. This is a big loss, and very likely this missing expert is one of the reasons for the 2001 seminal report from the Institute of Medicine (IOM) regarding mediation dosing errors: *"To Err Is Human,"* which noted that 98,000 people die each year as a result of preventable medical errors.[1] The number one error is medication dosing.

Yet medication errors continue to this day, with multiple authors noting that on the twentieth anniversary of the IOM publication, medical errors are still prevalent.[2] What we do know is that pharmacists are often the missing piece in the puzzle. The Agency for Healthcare Research and Quality reported that community pharmacists are a vital linchpin in decreasing medication errors,[3] more so than those obnoxiously ubiquitous alerts that pop up on our electronic health records. A pharmacist's guidance is nuanced, considers the patient wants/needs, cost and availability, the disease state, and the other competing medications and is the ultimate in "*patient-centered care*" that we all hold to be vitally important.

Physician Assist Clin 8 (2023) xv–xvi
https://doi.org/10.1016/j.cpha.2022.12.002

Thus, we are thrilled that Rebecca Maxson, PharmD and Professor of Pharmacy at Auburn University in Alabama, put together this issue of expert guidance from colleagues all over the United States. Please enjoy learning from the experts.

Kim Zuber, PAC, MS
131 31st Avenue North
St Petersburg, FL 33704, USA

Jane S. Davis, CRNP, DNP
University of Alabama at Birmingham
728 Richard Arrington, Boulevard South
Birmingham, AL 35233, USA

E-mail addresses:
zuberkim@yahoo.com (K. Zuber)
jsdavis@uabmc.edu (J.S. Davis)

REFERENCES

1. Institute of Medicine (US) Committee on Quality of Health Care in America. In: Kohn LT, Corrigan JM, Donaldson MS, editors. To err is human: building a safer health system. Washington, DC: National Academies Press (US); 2000. PMID: 25077248.
2. Dzau VJ, Shine KI. Two decades since to err is human: progress, but still a "chasm". JAMA 2020;324(24):2489–90.
3. Luchen GG, Hall KK, Hough KR. The role of community pharmacists in patient safety. Agency for Healthcare Research and Quality. Available at: https://psnet.ahrq.gov/perspective/role-community-pharmacists-patient-safety. Accessed November 8, 2022.

Preface
Medications: Do Good and Avoid Bad

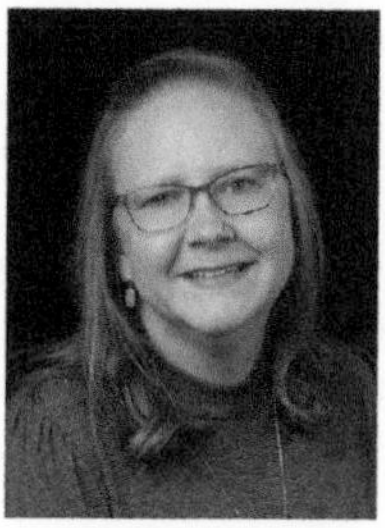

Rebecca Maxson, PharmD, BCPS
Editor

Pharmacology is a word of Latin origin, with -ology meaning the study of something and pharma referring to medications. Thus, pharmacology relates to the uses, effects, and modes of action of drugs.[1] In today's modern world, the appropriate use of medications (ie, drugs) is key to the health and well-being of our patients. Per the Centers for Disease Control and Prevention (CDC), from 2015 to 2018, 860 million medications were prescribed with 48.6% of Americans using at least one prescription medication in the past 30 days and with 12.8% using five or more in the past 30 days.[2] This represents about 9.2% (roughly 3.3 trillion US dollars) of the total health expenditures for 2018.[3]

Why so many medications? Due to the high burden of chronic diseases, all of which are treated with medications. In 2018, 51.8% of Americans older than 17 years of age had one chronic condition, with 27.2% having two or more chronic conditions.[4] These chronic conditions include arthritis, cancer, heart disease, lung disease, diabetes, hypertension, stroke, and kidney disease. All these disease states reduce our patients' quality and length of lives. In this issue, appropriate use of medications is discussed along with information to assist prescribers in understanding access issue for medications.

Davis begins our journey with an in-depth discussion on the history of medications and the pharmacy profession. Germain and Osmonsson provide a comprehensive discussion of treatment for heart failure, which affects about 6.2 million American adults.[5] Since on average an American has a stroke every 40 seconds,[5] stroke management during both the acute and the maintenance phases is explained by Starr and Trott. Treatment of hypertension is presented in two articles: first, Harlan and Farrer describe treating patients acutely with hypertensive crisits, and then Boyle and Remer provide excellent information on chronic hypertension management with many clinical pearls.

Physician Assist Clin 8 (2023) xvii–xix
https://doi.org/10.1016/j.cpha.2022.12.001

Smithgall provides a broad overview of medications used to treat common gastrointestinal diseases. Sewell and Johnson discuss up-to-date evidence for treating diabetes. The last chronic disease state management is kidney disease, with Salama, Sica, and Cardone providing key information on medications used to treat the various aspects of this disease that affects 14.8% of Americans.[5] They also provide an insightful discussion on adjusting medication doses in patients with reduced kidney function.

Prince provides excellent information on how to navigate the challenges of pain management during the current opioid epidemic, including an in-depth discussion of the risks and benefits of opioids and how to apply the recent CDC guidelines. As more states enact laws allowing for the medicinal use of marijuana, Hajjar provides the current evidence for the use of marijuana and explains the difference in medicinal marijuana and the ubiquitous CBD products.

An emerging field within medicine is the application of genetics in the diagnosis and treatment of individual patients. Kilpatrick, Givens, and Alexander have written an exceptional article including a pharmacogenetics primer and summary of current evidence for genetic variations and medication prescribing. This article is a must-read for all practitioners.

In 2020, 16.63% of the US population was over 65 years of age,[6] with 29% using at least five prescription medications.[7] Valentine and Hutchison present tips and information on how to optimize medication use in this vulnerable population.

In order to receive the mortality and morbidity benefit from medications, patients must have access to them. Zmajevac and McDowell explain the intricacies of insurance coverage for medications as well as the regulatory processes for both prescription medications and natural products.

Rebecca Maxson, PharmD, BCPS
Department of Pharmacy Practice
Auburn University Harrison College of Pharmacy
3720 Crossings Crest
Birmigham, AL 35242, USA

E-mail address:
maxsora@auburn.edu

REFERENCES

1. Merriam-Webster. Pharmacology. Available at: https://www.merriam-webster.com/dictionary/pharmacology. Accessed June 23, 2022.
2. CDC National Center for Health Statistics. Therapeutic drug use. Available at: https://www.cdc.gov/nchs/fastats/drug-use-therapeutic.htm. Accessed June 19, 2022.
3. CDC National Center for Health Statistics. Health Expenditures. Available at: https://www.cdc.gov/nchs/fastats/health-expenditures.htm. Accessed June 19, 2022.
4. Boersma P, Black LI, Ward BW. Prevalence of multiple chronic conditions among US adults, 2018. Prev Chronic Dis 2020;17:200130. https://doi.org/10.5888/pcd17.200130.
5. Virani SS, Alonso A, Benjamin EJ, et al. Heart disease and stroke statistics–2020 update: a report from the American Heart Association. Circulation 2020;141(9):e139–596.
6. Statista. Age distribution in the United States from 2010 to 2020. Available at: https://www.statista.com/statistics/270000/age-distribution-in-the-united-states/#:

~:text=In%202020%2C%20about%2018.37%20percent,over%2065%20years%20of%20age. Accessed June 23, 2022.
7. Qato DM, Alexander GC, Conti RM, et al. Use of prescription and over-the-counter medications and dietary supplements among older adults in the United States. J Am Med Assoc 2008;300:2867–78.

Pharmacy Through the Ages

From Potions to Patents

Jane S. Davis, CRNP, DNP

KEYWORDS

• Apothecary • Pharmacy • Compounding

KEY POINTS

- Humans have always depended on medications and ointments to treat various conditions and maladies.
- Over time, pharmacy has evolved as a profession separate from the practice of medicine.
- Today's pharmacist is essential to the health care team and is involved from research to delivery of care.

Humans have always looked to nature for survival. From nature, we feed, clothe, and shelter ourselves. Nature provides fuel for our transportation, our homes and buildings and even this journal. What often overlooked is that nature provides cures and treatments for common and not-so-common illnesses and for the prevention of future ailments. Think of the Roman soldier chewing willow bark for a headache; this was an early use of aspirin for pain relief. The foxglove plant, which beautifully graces summer gardens, produces digoxin, a lifesaving cardiac drug.

However, where did it begin? Who were the first pharmacists and what were they called? How were they trained? What was in their bag of remedies?

These questions will remain unanswered. Even the origin of the word pharmacist is obscure. A quick Internet search will come up with Latin and Greek words meaning anything from charm to cure to poison. Pharmacists themselves have had different titles over the years ranging from herbalist to healer to apothecaries, and even sorcerer or witch doctor. Regardless of the title, we have always looked to this profession for advice and dispensing of salves, ointments, pills, capsules, liquids, and vapors for our benefit. Whether an illness or condition was caused by bad humors, angry or evil spirits, or divine retribution, a solution could be found in a potion or application.

Pharmacy as a profession is both new and old. The first public pharmacy dates back to eighth century Baghdad.[1] Evidence of plants used as drugs dates back to prehistoric times with evidence found in caves.[2] The Egyptians were well versed in the use of medicinal cures. The *Ebers* Papyrus (1550 BC) listed approximately 800 prescriptions.[3]

Division of Nephrology, University of Alabama at Birmingham, 728 Richard Arrington boulevard S, Birmingham, AL 35233, USA
E-mail address: jsdavis@uabmc.edu

Physician Assist Clin 8 (2023) 237–241
https://doi.org/10.1016/j.cpha.2022.10.004

Ingredients included mustard, fig, myrrh, bat droppings, turtle shell powder, river silt, snakeskin, and "hair from the stomach of a cow." These ingredients were often dissolved in wine, beer, or milk, most likely to make them more palpable.[4]

In Asia, evidence of the use of prescriptions dates back to the first century AD. The Greeks who followed Hippocrates promoted life style changes and dietary modifications over drugs. All illnesses were thought to have their basis in the imbalance among the 4 elements—earth, air, fire, and water—and their relationship to the 4 humors—black bile, yellow bile, blood, and phlegm. Thus, conditions in which these elements were misaligned caused illness. Astrology also played a part in diagnosing and treating.

Galen in the second century did not disregard these elements. Instead, he promoted using drugs of a contrary nature to restore balance. Thus, something that was cool and wet might be applied to counteract an inflammation.

Unfortunately, during the European Middle Ages (roughly 400 AD to the mid-1400s) much of the knowledge gained was unavailable to the medical community because it was often written in Greek, which was not universally understood. In addition, church doctrine held that disease was the consequence of sin. However, at the same time, medical knowledge flourished in the Islamic world.

The printing press (1436) opened a new world for those who studied plants and their uses. Now someone in the possession of a book could identify a plant and utilize its healing properties. The exploration of the world outside of Europe brought new plants and herbs to be applied to various conditions.

Although there was little formal organization, pharmacists established guilds much like those of the Middle Ages. These guilds established rules for training new pharmacists and requirements before they were allowed to open shops. The guilds also regulated the numbers and locations of shops.

There was concern for the lack of standardization. Physicians wanted assurance that what they ordered from one shop would be prepared the same way in all shops. Although several pharmacopeias existed, the one considered to be the first was in 1546, the *Valerius Cordus*, in Nuremberg, Germany.[3]

Until the sixteenth and seventeenth centuries, in England, physicians were university educated, whereas apothecaries received their training in apprenticeships and practiced both medicine and pharmacy. Control of medications came under the purview of chemists and druggists. Instructions for use included crushing, infusing, boiling, filtering, and applying herbs and plants to affect a cure. At the same time, apothecary and chemistry were considered to be closely related. Johann Hartman, a trained apothecary, was the first professor of medical and pharmaceutical chemistry at the University of Marburg in 1609.

Pharmacy, chemistry, and medicine were often a chaotic mix with no locus of control. The advancement and professionalization of pharmacy as a profession defies a pattern. In the 1800s, in some parts of Europe, a successful pharmacist was one who was financially successful. Laws setting standards of practice as well as numbers and locations of pharmacies were passed to assure financial success for the pharmacist.

In England, however, it was much different. Pharmacists and apothecaries were substitute physicians and provided care for those who could not afford physicians. The definitions of who was a physician, apothecary, chemist, or druggist were fluid.

In the New World, the pioneer spirit and hope for a better life was attractive to many but there was little on the continent to attract medical practitioners. Given the low rates of literacy, few in the populace could read books on herbs and remedies. Medical care was provided by the educated in the community, often ministers or political leaders who, although literate, knew very little about medicine or pharmacology. As the colonies became more settled and urban, there were more professionals but often the physicians themselves managed the dispensaries where drugs were compounded and sold.

At this time, medications were not standardized, or mass produced. Patent medicines were the order of the day and widely available from many sources including peddlers or local bookstores. Early pharmacists often relied on compound recipes handed down within families. Rather than dispensing to the general public, they filled chests for physicians and landowners who in turn diagnosed, prescribed, and treated.[5]

The first known hospital pharmacist in the United States was Jonathan Roberts who was employed by the Pennsylvania Hospital in the 1750s. His duties included hospital rounds, compounding, and managing the hospital accounts and library. By the early part of the nineteenth century, pharmacists were regular fixtures in hospitals. In the early 1800s, New York Hospital required their pharmacist to pass an examination, provide references, and pay a US$250 bond attesting willingness to not abandon the post.[5]

Later in the nineteenth century, there was a movement to separate the practices of medicine and pharmacy. This, however, met with opposition because consumers saw they were paying both a physician and a pharmacist. Physicians, similarly, objected to losing revenue from acting as their own pharmacists.

The lines between the 2 professions often blurred because some physicians had "shops" in their offices that included compounded products, patent medicines, and often sundries. These physicians would frequently hire drug clerks or apothecaries to dispense medications. At the time, pharmacology was not a regular part of medical training.[5] In the 1870s, laws were passed that managed the practice of pharmacy.[3]

The date and location of America's first drugstore is unclear. New Orleans lays claim for having the first because it was opened by a registered pharmacist. However, Fredericksburg, VA, also claims to be the site of first drug store naming Mrs. George Washington as one of its patrons.[6,7]

The relationship between physicians and pharmacists continued to be fluid, vacillating between cooperation and competition. On one hand, during the 1800s, pharmacists relieved the physicians of the tasks of compounding their own drugs. With many products coming from different areas, it was often up to the pharmacist to attest to the purity and potency of a product. On the other hand, some apothecaries were filling prescriptions without a physician order, revising prescriptions, or treating patients on their own.[3]

Pharmacy education was moving away from apprenticeships and into the universities. The first formal pharmacy school, *Philadelphia College of Pharmacy*, opened in 1821, and in 1852, the American Pharmaceutical Association was founded.[6] Initially, the classes were taught at night because most students worked as clerks and apprentices during the day. Each student was required to attend every lecture 2 times, write an article, and pass a test. At the end, students were awarded a diploma. Despite more than 20 years of educating pharmacists, it was not until 1846 that the Philadelphia College of Pharmacy hired its first true pharmacy professor, William J Procter, Jr, who is known as the Father of American Pharmacy.[5]

In the twentieth century, the role of the pharmacist and physician separated and became more defined with physicians growing in their role of diagnosing and treating and the pharmacist continuing the compounding and safe dispensing of medications ordered by the physician. At this time, the corner drug store was a staple of American life. Often presided over by a pharmacist, it still contained and dispensed medications but in addition, often had a soda fountain and a tobacco counter, which were often more profitable than the dispensary. The pharmacist behind the counter dispensing medications and sodas is the picture most Americans had of the pharmacist.

The 1906 Food and Drugs Act (FDA) passed the US Congress primarily to assure the safety of food. However, it also addressed many issues confronting the practice of pharmacy. These included the use of patent medications whose ingredients were often questionable and whose efficacy was even more so. With these rules and the development of mass production, medication production began to be the purview of the pharmaceutical industry. In the 1930s, approximately 75% prescriptions were compounded by pharmacists; by 1970, that was only 1%.[3] Growth of the pharmaceutical industry was driven by several factors including increased medical research after World War II, population boom after World War II and the increase in standard of living. From 1930 to 2013, the number of FDA-approved new medical entities (ie, new drugs) increased to 1453 with the largest growth seen in the 1980s to 2010s.[8]

With the emergence of the pharmaceutical industry and movement from pharmacist-compounding medications to dispensing mass-produced medications, the pharmacy profession began moving from a product-oriented to a patient-oriented profession.[9] Evidence of this change was the addition of a Doctor of Pharmacy (PharmD) degree to the Bachelor of Science in Pharmacy (BS Pharm) in the 1950s. By the 1970s, the PharmD degree was available at most schools and colleges of pharmacy. In 1997, the pharmacy education accrediting body announced that they would stop accrediting BS Pharm degrees starting in 2000, thus resulting in the PharmD degree being the only option available today. In parallel to the rise of the PharmD degree, postgraduate (PG) residencies started in the 1960s. These early residencies focused on leadership skills in pharmacy administration and traditional pharmacy operations.[9] Subsequent programs added clinical pharmacy activities to these traditional roles.

Paralleling the education and PG residency training, the 1950s saw the beginning of clinical pharmacy practice in the United States. The pharmacy profession changed due to the increase in available medications, patients and providers needed a drug-therapy expert who understands the mechanism of action, adverse effects, drug interactions, dosing, and role in therapy for the increasing numbers of available medications.[10] Additionally, in the 1950s and 1960s, the institution of Medicare and Medicaid increased access to health care while the veterans from World War II were aging and requiring more extensive care in the Veterans Administration System.[9] All of these factors were opportunities for pharmacists to assist more directly in patient care.

The earliest clinical activities were the emergence of drug information centers at universities and academic medical centers.[9] The implementation of unit dose services allowed pharmacists in hospitals to be closer to the bedside where they could interact more directly with physicians and nurses. Although hospital clinical pharmacy was growing, the advent of pharmacists in ambulatory practices was also occurring with early growth in the management of warfarin.[9]

Today, clinical pharmacists are the drug experts who round in hospitals, teach in schools and colleges of pharmacy, and provide care alongside physicians and advanced practitioners. Additionally, they liaise with and support community pharmacists who are still ensuring safe medication dispensing while also providing patient counseling, recommendations for over-the-counter products and providing Medication Therapy Management services.

Over the centuries, the role of the pharmacist has evolved and grown with that of other medical professions. Once trained by an apothecary with little to no formal education, the University-based PharmD degree is now required as entry level to the profession. Many graduates further their education by enrolling in residency programs to gain more experience in a particular aspect of pharmacy.

The pharmacist of the past who counted tablets and measured liquids is fast disappearing. However, the need for pharmacists with their specialized training and knowledge of the science of medications, how they act and interact with other medications has never been greater. Adverse drug events are a leading cause of death in the United States, and pharmacists, with their knowledge, are in a perfect position to intervene.

More than 100 years later, the Bachelor Degree in Pharmacy became the entry level standard followed in 1997 by the PharmD.

CLINICS CARE POINTS

- Pharmacy has evolved along side with medicine to deliver high quality, modern health care
- The future of pharmacy is not static and the pharmacist of the future may well be a part of the diagnostic and treatment of patients.

DISCLOSURE

No disclosures relevant to this article.

REFERENCES

1. Kheir N, Zaiden M, Younes H, et al. Pharmacy education and practice in 13 middle eastern countries. Am J Pharm Educ 2008;72(6):133.
2. Hardy K. Paleomedicine and the evolutionary context of medicinal plant use. Rev Bras Farmacogn 2021;31(1):1–15. Accessed March 15, 22.
3. Higby GJ. Evolution of pharmacy. Chapter 2 in remington: the science and practice of pharmacy. 22nd ed. Pharmaceutical Press; 2013. p. 11–24.
4. The History of Pharmacy. Texas tech university health. Available at: https://www.ttuhsc.edu: pharmacy museum. Accessed Feb 27, 22.
5. Higby GJ. From compounding to caring: an abridged history of american pharmacy. In: Knowlton C, Penna R, editors. Pharmaceutical care. NY: Chapman and Hall; 1996. p. pp18–45. Chapter 2.
6. Available at: https://www.drugstoremuseum.com/drugstore. Accessed April 28, 22.
7. Gebhart F. Going beyond dispensing: the future of pharmacist roles. Drug Top J March 2020;164:3. https://www.drugtopics.com. Accessed 1 May 2022.
8. Kinch MS, Haynesworth A, Kinch SL, et al. An overview of FDA-approved new molecular entities: 1827-2013. Drug Discov Today 2014;19:1033–9.
9. Carter B. Evolution of clinical pharmacy in the USA and future directions for patient care. Drugs Aging 2016;33:169–77.
10. Miller R. History of clinical pharmacy and clinical pharmacology. J Clin Pharmacol 1981;21:195–7.

Medications for When the Heart Fails

Kenda E. Germain, PharmD, BCPS*, Alyssa J. Osmonson, PharmD, BCPS

KEYWORDS

- Heart failure • Heart failure with reduced ejection fraction
- Guideline-directed medical therapy

KEY POINTS

- Heart failure with reduced ejection fraction (HFrEF) is a chronic disease carrying a significant public health burden.
- Despite long-standing availability of life-saving and morbidity limiting treatment options, there remains a consistent underutilization of guideline-directed medical therapy (GDMT).
- All patients with a diagnosis of HFrEF should be initiated on an angiotensin II receptor blocker with neprilysin inhibitor (preferred), angiotensin-converting enzyme inhibitor, or angiotensin receptor blocker, plus an evidence-based beta-blocker, titrated to target or maximum tolerated doses.
- Patients should be assessed for addition of other appropriate GDMT, with choice of agents driven by patient-specific factors.

INTRODUCTION

Heart failure (HF) carries a significant public health burden, affecting patients, caregivers, providers, and health care systems. Compounding this, prevalence is escalating rapidly in the United States (US), with nearly 1 million new HF diagnoses made annually, and a national prevalence of more than 6 million American adults.[1,2] Unfortunately, these numbers are projected to worsen with the aging population projected to drive an increase in HF prevalence of 46% by the year 2030, which will cause additional strain on the health care system and disease burden for patients and their families.[3] HF is an overarching term encompassing both HF with reduced ejection fraction (HFrEF), formerly congestive HF, and HF with preserved ejection fraction (HFpEF). HFrEF is defined as a clinical diagnosis of HF and a left ventricular ejection fraction (LVEF) ≤40%, whereas HFpEF is a clinical diagnosis of HF with an LVEF greater than 40%. Cases in the United States are relatively evenly split with about 53% of patients diagnosed with HFrEF and 47% with HFpEF, although gender and

Department of Pharmacy Birmingham, Princeton Baptist Medical Center Birmingham, 701 Princeton Avenue Southwest, Birmingham, AL 35211, USA
* Corresponding author.
E-mail address: kenda.germain@bhsala.com

Physician Assist Clin 8 (2023) 243–258
https://doi.org/10.1016/j.cpha.2022.10.005
physicianassistant.theclinics.com

racial disparities consistent with heart disease as a whole hold true with black men and white women disproportionately affected.[2] In addition to the high prevalence of HF, it also carries a remarkably high mortality risk, with a 5-year mortality rate over 52% and 1-year mortality rate of almost 30%.[3]

Despite long-standing availability of life-saving and morbidity limiting treatment options, there remains a consistent underutilization of guideline-directed medical therapy (GDMT). Alternatively, there are limited disease-modifying pharmacotherapy options for patients with HFpEF, making its treatment aims less well-defined.[4] Recently, evolving evidence has revealed opportunities to change the progression of the disease by combining therapies to improve morbidity and mortality outcomes and quality of life for patients with chronic HFrEF, which will be the focus of this review.[5,6]

HFrEF is classified using the American College of Cardiology/American Heart Association (ACC/AHA) Stages of HF. Stages range A through D, with Stage A being high risk for HF but without structural heart disease or symptoms of HF and Stage D being refractory HF requiring specialized interventions[6] (**Table 1**). HFrEF is further defined using the New York Heart Association (NYHA) functional classification criteria ranging from Class I to Class IV, with Class I having no limitation of physical activity and Class IV unable to perform any physical activity without symptoms of HF or symptoms of HF at rest[6] (**Table 2**).

Established pharmacotherapy options for chronic HFrEF include angiotensin II receptor blocker with neprilysin inhibitors (ARNIs), angiotensin-converting enzyme inhibitors (ACEIs), angiotensin receptor blockers (ARBs), beta-blockers (BBs), mineralocorticoid receptor antagonists (MRAs, formerly known as aldosterone antagonists), loop diuretics, sodium–glucose cotransporter 2 (SGLT2) inhibitors, hydralazine/isosorbide dinitrate, ivabradine, digoxin, and vericiguat (**Table 3**). These agents have been shown in randomized controlled trials (RCTs) to improve symptoms, reduce hospitalizations, and/or prolong survival. Optimal therapy is defined as treatment provided at either the target or highest-tolerated dose for a given patient, with target doses being the doses targeted in clinical trials[6] (**Table 4**).

Patients should be initiated on GDMT promptly on diagnosis of HFrEF. Recommendations for initiating GDMT in patients with newly diagnosed symptomatic HFrEF (NYHA Stage C) are reviewed in **Fig. 1**.[6] In regard to which agent to initiate first, the ACC/AHA guidelines recommend initiating an inhibitor of the renin-angiotensin-aldosterone system (RAAS), including ARNI, ACEI, or ARB or an evidence-based BB (carvedilol, metoprolol, or bisoprolol) first.[6] Whichever is chosen should be uptitrated to the target or maximum tolerated doses in a timely fashion (ie, every 2 weeks). Patient-specific factors such as predominant symptoms ("wet" vs "dry"), kidney function, serum potassium levels, and resting heart rate should be considered when choosing an initial agent. BB should not be initiated in patients with signs or symptoms of decompensated HF.[6] Agents should then be added and titrated to target dose as able to optimize GDMT HFrEF treatment.

GUIDELINE-DIRECTED MEDICAL THERAPY

Angiotensin II Receptor Blocker with Neprilysin Inhibitor

ARNIs are a combination drug consisting of a neprilysin inhibitor and an ARB. Neprilysin inhibitors are prodrugs that inhibit neprilysin, an endopeptidase that degrades several endogenous vasoactive peptides, leading to increased levels of peptides, including natriuretic peptides, bradykinin, and adrenomedullin. Increasing the levels of these substrates counteracts neurohormonal over activation that contributes to vasoconstriction, sodium retention, and maladaptive remodeling.[7,8] Because

Table 1
The American College of Cardiology/American Heart Association Stages of heart failure

Stage	*Criteria*	*Description*	*Symptoms*	*Worsens A → D with Disease Progression*
A	At high risk for HF but without structural heart disease or symptoms of HF	• Called pre-heart failure • Includes patients with HTN, diabetes, CAD, and metabolic syndrome, those using cardiotoxins, and those with a family history of cardiomyopathy	Do not experience symptoms	
B	Structural heart disease but without signs or symptoms of HF	• Still pre-heart failure • Can be caused by previous MI, LV remodeling including LVH and low EF, or valvular disease	Do not experience symptoms, but may have an enlarged left ventricle affecting the hearts ability to pump effectively	
C	Structural heart disease with prior or current symptoms of HF	Underlying structural disease affects the left ventricle's contraction function	Common symptoms: • SOB • Fatigue • Anginal pain	
D	Refractory HF requiring specialized interventions	• Advanced or end-stage HF • Often with recurrent hospitalization despite GDMT	Significant symptoms during physical activity and at rest, even when receiving treatment, include • Swelling • Persistent cough • PND • Cognitive change	

Abbreviations: ACC, American College of Cardiology; AHA, American Heart Association; CAD, coronary artery disease; EF, ejection fraction; GDMT, guideline-directed medical therapy; HF, heart failure; HTN, hypertension; LV, left ventricular; LVH, left ventricular hypertrophy; MI, myocardial infarction, PND, paroxysmal nocturnal dyspnea; SOB, shortness of breath.

Table 2
New York Heart Association functional classification

Functional Classification	*Criteria*	*Description*	*Symptoms*	*Variable I → IV Based on Symptom Control and Disease Progression*
Class I	No limitation of physical activity	Ordinary physical activity does not cause symptoms of HF	None	
Class II	Slight limitation of physical activity	Comfortable at rest, but ordinary physical activity results in symptoms of HF	• Palpitations • Fatigue • SOB	
Class III	Marked limitation of physical activity	Comfortable at rest, but less than ordinary activity causes symptoms of HF	• Fatigue • SOB • Anginal pain	
Class IV	HF symptoms present with any activity, and even at rest	Unable to perform any physical activity without symptoms of HF, or symptoms of HF at rest	• Swelling • Persistent cough • PND • Cognitive change	

NYHA = New York Heart Association; HF = heart failure; SOB = shortness of breath; PND = paroxysmal nocturnal dyspnea

Table 3
Drug class review

Drug Class	Mechanism of Action	Adverse Effects	Monitoring Parameters	Pearls/ Clinical Considerations
ARNI	Neprilysin inhibitor (induces vasodilation and natriuresis) + ARB (inhibition of AT2 type 1 receptor)	• Hypotension • Hyperkalemia • AKI • Angioedema	• K • SCr • BP	• Works on RAAS compensatory mechanism • First-line agent • Mortality benefit • If previously on ACEI, need 36 hour off before initiation
ACEIs	Competitive inhibitor of ACE leading to reduction in conversion of AT1 to AT2	• Hypotension • Hyperkalemia • AKI • Drug cough • Angioedema (rare)	• K • SCr • BP • Reported cough	• "-prils" • Works on RAAS compensatory mechanism • Consider when ARNI not tolerated/cost prohibitive • Mortality benefit
ARBs	Inhibition of the AT2 type 1 receptor	• Hypotension • Hyperkalemia • AKI	• K • SCr • BP	• "-sartans" • Works on RAAS compensatory mechanism • Consider when ARNI not tolerated/cost prohibitive • Mortality benefit
β-blockers	Inhibition of beta-adrenergic receptors ± alpha adrenergic activity	• Bradycardia • Hypotension • Dizziness	• HR • BP	• "-lols" • Evidence based BBs: carvedilol, metoprolol succinate, or bisoprolol • Mortality benefit
Loop diuretics	Inhibits reabsorption of Na and Cl in the kidney (loop of Henle), causing a natriuretic effect	• Hypotension • Dizziness • Frequent urination • Muscle cramps • Thirst	• Volume status • SCr • Electrolytes • BP • Urine output	• For patients with persistent volume overload • Symptom management • Dosing may be guided by (fluid-driven) changes in weight

(*continued on next page*)

Table 3
(continued)

Drug Class	Mechanism of Action	Adverse Effects	Monitoring Parameters	Pearls/ Clinical Considerations
Mineralocorticoid receptor antagonists	Inhibition of aldosterone receptor increasing NaCl and water excretion while conserving K and hydrogen ions	• Hyperkalemia • Worsening renal function • Gynecomastia (spironolactone)	• K • SCr	• "Potassium-sparing diuretic" ↑ Na, Cl, and water excretion, while conserving K ions • Works on RAAS compensatory mechanism • Mortality benefit
SGLT2 inhibitors	Inhibition of SGLT2, reducing Na reabsorption, which may decrease cardiac preload/ afterload and downregulate sympathetic activity	• AKI • Genital mycotic infection and/or UTI • Hypoglycemia • Ketoacidosis • Dyslipidemia	• BMP/SCr • HbA1c • BP • Glucose • Volume status	• "-gliflozins" • Mortality benefit • Check minimum renal function requirements prior to initiation
Nitrates	Increased cGMP concentration resulting in smooth muscle contraction	• HA • Dizziness • Hypotension	BP	• Example: isosorbide dinitrate • Used in combination with hydralazine (individually dosed or as fixed combination) • Consider for persistently symptomatic Black patients despite GDMT
Hydralazine	Direct vasodilation of arterioles resulting in decreased systemic resistance	• HA • Dizziness • Hypotension	BP	• Used in combination with isosorbide dinitrate (individually dosed or as fixed combination) • Consider for persistently symptomatic Black patients despite GDMT
Ivabradine	Inhibition of the If channels in the SA node leading to prolonged diastolic depolarization and reduced HR	• Bradycardia • AF	• HR • Heart rhythm	• Reduces risk of hospitalization with stable HF with HR ≥70 BPM on maximally tolerated BB • Patient needs to be in NSR • Contraindicated in AF

Table 3
(continued)

Drug Class	Mechanism of Action	Adverse Effects	Monitoring Parameters	Pearls/ Clinical Considerations
Digoxin	Inhibition of Na/K channel resulting in increased intracellular calcium and contractility	• GI upset (nausea/ vomiting) • Visual disturbances • Lethargy • Arrhythmias	• Digoxin serum concentration • HR • Heart rhythm	• Reduces risk of hospitalization and leads to improvement in symptoms and exercise tolerance • Requires monitoring of levels • Watch for drug interactions
Vericiguat	Enhances production of cGMP leading to smooth muscle relaxation and vasodilation	• Hypotension • Anemia	• BP • CBC	• For patients with progression of HFrEF despite GDMT • Reduces hospitalization and cardiovascular death • cGMP has potential for improving HF via vasodilation, improvement in endothelial function, and decreasing fibrosis and remodeling of the heart

Abbreviations: ACEI, angiotensin-converting enzyme inhibitor; AF, atrial fibrillation; AKI, acute kidney injury; ARB, angiotensin receptor blocker; ARNI, angiotensin II receptor blocker with neprilysin inhibitors; AT1, angiotensin I; AT2, angiotensin II; BB, beta-blocker; BMP, basic metabolic panel; BP, blood pressure; CBC, complete blood count; cGMP, cyclic guanosine monophosphate; Cl, chloride; GDMT, guideline-directed medical therapy; GI, gastrointestinal; HA, headache; HbA1c, hemoglobin A1c; HF, heart failure; HFrEF, heart failure with reduced ejection fraction; HR, heart rate; K, potassium, Na, sodium; NSR, normal sinus rhythm; RAAS, renin-angiotensin-aldosterone system; SA, sinoatrial; SCr, serum creatinine; SGLT2, sodium–glucose cotransporter 2; UTI, urinary tract infection.

Table 4
Starting and target doses of medication therapies for HFrEF (Stage C)

	Starting Dose	Target Dose
ARNI		
Sacubitril/valsartan	49–51 mg twice daily	97/103 mg twice daily
ACEIs		
Captopril	6.25 mg three times daily	50 mg three times daily
Enalapril	2.5 mg twice daily	10–20 mg twice daily
Lisinopril	2.5–5 mg daily	20–40 mg daily
Ramipril	1.2 mg daily	10 mg daily
ARBs		
Candesartan	4–8 mg daily	32 mg daily
Losartan	25–50 mg daily	150 mg daily
Valsartan	40 mg twice daily	160 mg twice daily
Beta-Blockers		
Bisoprolol	1.25 mg once daily	10 mg once daily
Carvedilol	3.125 mg twice daily	<85 kg: 25 mg twice daily ≥85 kg: 50 mg twice daily
Metoprolol succinate	12.5–25 mg daily	200 mg daily
Mineralocorticoid Receptor Antagonist		
Eplerenone	25 mg daily	50 mg daily
Spironolactone	12.5–25 mg daily	25–50 mg daily
SGLT2i		
Dapagliflozin	10 mg daily	10 mg daily
Empagliflozin	10 mg daily	10 mg daily
Vasodilators		
Hydralazine	25 mg three times daily	100 mg three times daily
Isosorbide dinitrate	20–30 mg three times daily	40 mg three times daily
If Channel Blocker		
Ivabradine	5 mg twice daily	7.5 mg twice daily
Additional agents		
Vericiguat	2.5 mg daily	10 mg daily
Digoxin	0.125–0.52 mg daily	Patient specific for target serum concentration of 0.5–0.9 ng/mL

Abbreviations: ACEI, angiotensin converting enzyme inhibitor; ARBs, angiotensin receptor blockers; ARNI, angiotensin-receptor neprilysin inhibitor; SGLT2, sodium–glucose cotransporter 2 inhibitor.

angiotensin II is also a substrate for neprilysin, neprilysin inhibitors raise angiotensin levels when coadministered with an ARB. ARBs produce direct antagonism of the angiotensin II (AT2) receptors, displacing AT2 from the AT1 receptor, and antagonize AT1-induced vasoconstriction, aldosterone release, catecholamine release, arginine vasopressin release, water intake, and hypertrophic responses.[7,8] The only available ARNI in the United States is sacubitril/valsartan, which was tested in patients with chronic HFrEF in the PARADIGM-HF trial, an RCT looking at patients with NYHA class II through IV symptoms and an EF of ≤40% (adjusted to ≤35% 1 year into the trial) that were on stable doses of ACEIs or ARBs, and on other GDMT. PARADIGM-HF revealed an absolute 4.7% reduction in the primary outcome of cardiovascular (CV) death or HF

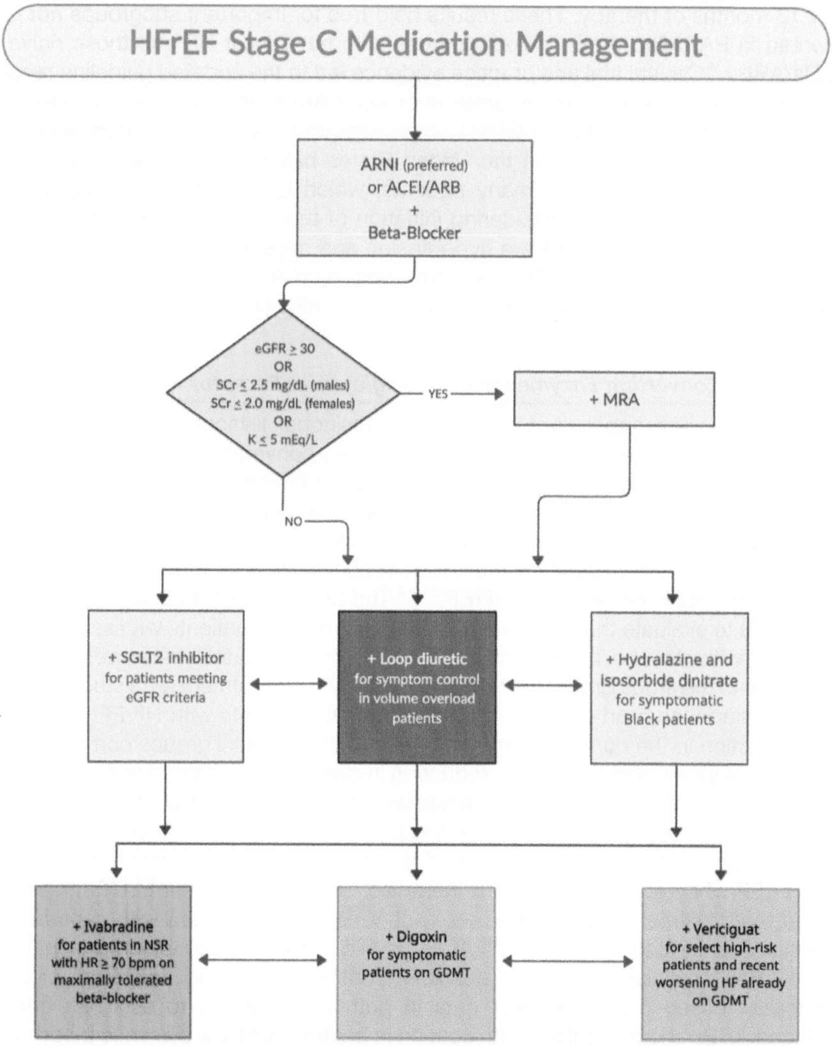

Fig. 1. Medication management. Blue = Class of recommendation (COR) 1, level of evidence (LOE) A; purple = COR 1, LOE B-NR; orange = COR 2a, LOE B-R; gold = COR 2b, LOE B-R. ACEI, angiotensin converting enzyme inhibitor; ARB, angiotensin receptor blocker; ARNI, angiotensin-neprilysn inhibitor; eGFR measured in mL/mL/min/1.73m^2; HFrEF, heart failure with reduced ejection fraction; K, potassium; MRA, mineralocorticoid receptor antagonist; SGLT2, sodium glucose cotransporter 2. (*Adapted from* Heidenreich P, Bozkurt B, Aguilar D, et al. 2022 AHA/ACC/HFSA Guideline for the Management of Heart Failure. J Am Coll Cardiol. 2022 May, 79 (17) e263–e421. https://doi.org/10.1016/j.jacc.2021.12.012.)

hospitalization and an absolute 2.8% reduction in death from any cause in patients treated with sacubitril/valsartan versus enalapril. Hypotension was more common in the study group, whereas reduction in kidney function was not. Angioedema was numerically higher in the study group, but not statistically different between groups. The trial was stopped early at 27 months based on reaching the prespecified boundary for an overwhelming benefit with sacubitril/valsartan.[8] In the PROVE-HF study, median LVEF increased from 28.2% to 37.8% (9.4% increase) in the sacubitril/valsartan group after 12 months of therapy. These results held true for important subgroups not represented in PARADIGM-HF, including those with new onset HF and those naive to ACEIs/ARBs.[9] Clinical trial and practice evidence led to the updated guideline recommendation placing ARNIs as preferred over ACEI/ARBs as initial therapy (direct-to-ARNI approach) or to optimize GDMT when tolerated and not cost-prohibitive. The only ARNI currently available in the United States has no generic option available, making it cost-prohibitive for many patients, which is an important consideration and potential barrier when considering initiation of therapy. The most common side effects associated with ANRIs are hypotension and hyperkalemia. Note, if switching from ACEI to ARNI, ensure a 36-h washout period off ACEI before initiation of ARNI to reduce the risk of angioedema.[8] No washout is required when switching from an ARB to ARNI.

Angiotensin-Converting Enzyme Inhibitor/Angiotensin Receptor Blocker

ACEIs, such as benazepril, captopril, enalapril, fosinopril, lisinopril, quinapril, and ramipril, work as a competitive inhibitor of angiotensin-converting enzyme (ACE), which prevents conversion of AT1 to AT2, a potent vasoconstrictor, resulting in lower levels of AT2 (similarly to ARBs) and an increase in plasma renin activity and a reduction in aldosterone secretion.[10] ACEI and ARBs have been shown to attenuate ventricular remodeling and improve ventricular function, reducing HF progression, hospitalization, and mortality rate in patients with HFrEF.[11,12] The CONSENSUS trial was the first landmark study to evaluate the effect of enalapril on mortality in patients with severe HFrEF compared with placebo. It demonstrated 6 and 12 month mortality rates were 40% and 31% lower in the study group, respectively.[13] SOLVD-T (treatment arm) studied the effect of enalapril on mortality and hospitalizations for patients with HFrEF revealing a 16% reduction in the cumulative mortality rate in the enalapril groups compared with placebo at 4 years, and a 26% risk reduction in death or hospitalization for worsening HF.[14] ARBs, such as candesartan, irbesartan, losartan, olmesartan, telmisartan, and valsartan have demonstrated similar findings. The CHARM study showed candesartan significantly reduced all-cause mortality, CV death, and HF hospitalizations in patients with HFrEF when added to standard therapies.[15] Furthermore, the ELITE II trial suggested that treatment with losartan was not superior to treatment with captopril but was significantly better tolerated.[16] ACEI or ARB should be considered in patients where ARNI administration is not possible (contraindicated, not tolerated, or cost-prohibitive) based on robust RCT data in both drug classes to establish benefit. ACEI and ARBs should be used with caution in patients with low systemic blood pressure, kidney disease, or elevated serum potassium.[6] Initial administration of ACEIs and ARBs is associated with a transient increase in serum creatinine, which typically stabilizes within the first few months of therapy. A rise of up to 30% is generally considered acceptable. Although both classes can cause angioedema, incidence is lower with ARBs than ACEIs. In addition, ARBs do not lead to bradykinin accumulation and therefore are not associated with cough like ACEIs.[10] Patients who experience hyperkalemia from an ACEI/ARB can be prescribed a potassium binder, so that they can remain on these medications (see Chapter 10, Medications for the Kidney, for more information). There are affordable options in both drug classes, including widespread coverage of at least one agent per class on all major prescription drug insurance plans, as well as free and $4 programs for un/underinsured patients at many retail pharmacies.

Beta-Blockers

BBs lead to inhibition of beta-adrenoreceptor (beta-selective) and alpha-adrenergic activity (for nonselective/mixed alpha-BBs), which blocks sympathetic nervous system activation, slowing left ventricular remodeling that would worsen myocardial function.[17–19] There are three evidence-based BBs: bisoprolol, carvedilol, and metoprolol succinate (extended release/XL).[18] The landmark trials investigating the evidence-based BB are CIBIS-II (bisoprolol), MERIT-HF (metoprolol succinate), and COPERNICUS (carvedilol), with all three demonstrating reduced all-cause mortality and hospitalization when combined with other GDMT, in various degrees of HF (mild to severe).[20–22] The reduction in mortality is not thought to be a class effect. Carvedilol, with its nonselective action, may be advantageous in patients with HFrEF experiencing hypertension versus bisoprolol or metoprolol, which have marginal blood pressure lowering effects.[18,19] Patients who are decompensated or hypervolemic at initiation are at higher risk of worsening HF, so BB should not be initiated until patients are compensated. Bradycardia, hypotension, and dizziness are the primarily observed side effects of BB therapy.[17] BBs are generally very affordable, with carvedilol and metoprolol succinate coming in slightly cheaper than bisoprolol for some patients depending on insurance coverage status.

Mineralocorticoid Receptor Antagonists

MRAs, including spironolactone and eplerenone, provide benefit in HF by competitive inhibition of aldosterone in the kidney's distal convoluted tubules, increasing sodium chloride and water excretion while conserving potassium, which is why these agents are also called potassium-sparing diuretics.[23] Clinical trials have demonstrated survival benefit when MRAs are used in addition to GDMT in patients with advanced HF (spironolactone in the RALES trial) and patients with mild HF symptoms (eplerenone in the EMPHASIS-HF trial).[24,25] Because of the findings from these studies, guidelines recommend MRAs should be used in patients with NYHA classes II–IV receiving GDMT with an eGFR $\geq$30 mL/min/1.72 m^2 or $\leq$ 2.5 mg/dL in males or $\leq$2 mg/dL in females and a K $\leq$ 5 mEq/L.[6] MRAs are generally well tolerated, with the primary adverse reaction leading to discontinuation being hyperkalemia.[24] Male patients on spironolactone had a significant increase in the development of gynecomastia, but this did not occur with eplerenone.[24,25]

Sodium–Glucose Cotransporter 2 Inhibitors

The SGLT2 inhibitors, canagliflozin, dapagliflozin, empagliflozin, and ertugliflozin, are routine agents used in managing diabetes. However, recent data have demonstrated positive benefits of SGLT2 inhibitors in patients with HFrEF in the presence and absence of diabetes. When comparing a SGLT2 inhibitor with placebo, there was a 25% reduction in the composite outcome of CV death or hospitalization due to HF in both the DAPA-HF and EMPEROR-Reduced trials.[5] In addition, there was greater than 30% reduction in HF-related hospitalizations. Dapagliflozin was associated with a statistically significant reduction in CV death and all-cause mortality, although CV mortality benefits were not observed with empagliflozin. It is important to note, only roughly 50% of patients in both the DAPA-HF and EMPEROR-Reduced trials had concomitant diabetes.[26,27] Although the mechanism for the benefit of SGLT2 inhibitors in HF is not fully understood, based on the clinical evidence it is not from their effects on blood glucose or osmotic diuresis. A theory on the mechanism is the interaction of SGLT2 inhibitors with sodium–hydrogen exchangers, which are responsible for most sodium tubular reuptake and whose activity is enhanced in patients with HFrEF. More specifically in the heart, SGLT2 inhibitors block sodium–hydrogen exchange, which results in reduced cardiac injury, hypertrophy, and remodeling.[28] Currently, only dapagliflozin and empagliflozin are FDA-approved for use in HFrEF. When initiating these agents ensure eGFR is > 30 mL/min/1.73 m^2 for dapagliflozin and greater than 20 mL/min/1.73 m^2 for empagliflozin. Adverse effects associated with SGLT2 inhibitors include genital mycotic infections and/or urinary tract infections, hypoglycemia, and ketoacidosis.[29,30] One should consider the patient's ability to obtain the medication when prescribing a SGLT2 inhibitor, as they are more expensive than other first-line agents depending on insurance.

ADDITIONAL TREATMENTS

Vasodilators

Hydralazine directly vasodilates the arterioles, with little effect on veins, whereas isosorbide dinitrate stimulates cyclic guanosine monophosphate (cGMP) resulting in relaxation of both arterial and venous smooth muscle, with a more prominent effect on veins. The V-HeFT trial assessed the effects of vasodilator therapy in chronic HF patients already receiving digoxin and diuretic therapy. Results included a statistically significant reduction in 2-year mortality of 34% compared with the addition of prazosin.[31] In addition, the combination of these agents has been shown to increase survival and symptom burden, specifically, in African American patients with HFrEF. In the A-HeFT trial, African American patients with NYHA class II or IV HF received fixed-dose hydralazine plus isosorbide dinitrate in addition to standard therapy versus placebo. The study was terminated early due to an increased rate of mortality in those receiving placebo. There was a 43% reduction in death from any cause and a 33% reduction in the rate of first hospitalization for HF observed.[32] The combination is currently recommended in African American patients receiving GDMT or in those who cannot tolerate first-line agents due to intolerance or kidney disease.[5] Vasodilators are commonly associated with headache, dizziness, edema, and hypotension.

Loop Diuretics

Loop diuretics, bumetanide, furosemide, and torsemide are the preferred diuretic agents in patients with HFrEF.[5] These agents exhibit their effect by inhibiting reabsorption of sodium and chloride in the ascending loop of Henle and the proximal convoluted tubule in the kidneys. The net result is an increase in water and electrolyte (calcium, chloride, magnesium, phosphate, and sodium) excretion.[33] Owing to their effects on sodium, and thus water excretion, loop diuretics have demonstrated a clear benefit in decreasing congestive symptoms and improving quality of life in patients with HFrEF. However, their utility in reducing morbidity and mortality has not been well demonstrated. Thus, loop diuretics should not be used in the absence of GDMT. When used in combination, these agents have been shown to reduce the occurrence of hospitalizations and prevent disease progression. Loop diuretics should be initiated at the standard starting dose and titrated to the lowest dose possible that results in euvolemia. Of important note, diuretic resistance can occur and can be combated by escalation of diuretic dose and/or the addition of an alternative diuretic agent.[5] Adverse effects of loop diuretics include hypotension, dizziness, hypokalemia, dehydration, and increased urinary frequency.[33] These agents are generally affordable and attainable for most patients.

Ivabradine

Heart rate is a strong predictor of CV outcomes in patients with HF, with an increased HR leading to adverse outcomes.[5] Ivabradine is an I_f channel inhibitor that works by blocking f-channels in the sinoatrial (SA) node resulting in a reduction in HR.[34] In the SHIFT trial, patients with symptomatic HF, an LVEF of $\leq$35%, in sinus rhythm with an HR of $\geq$70 bpm, hospitalized within the last year, and receiving GDMT, including

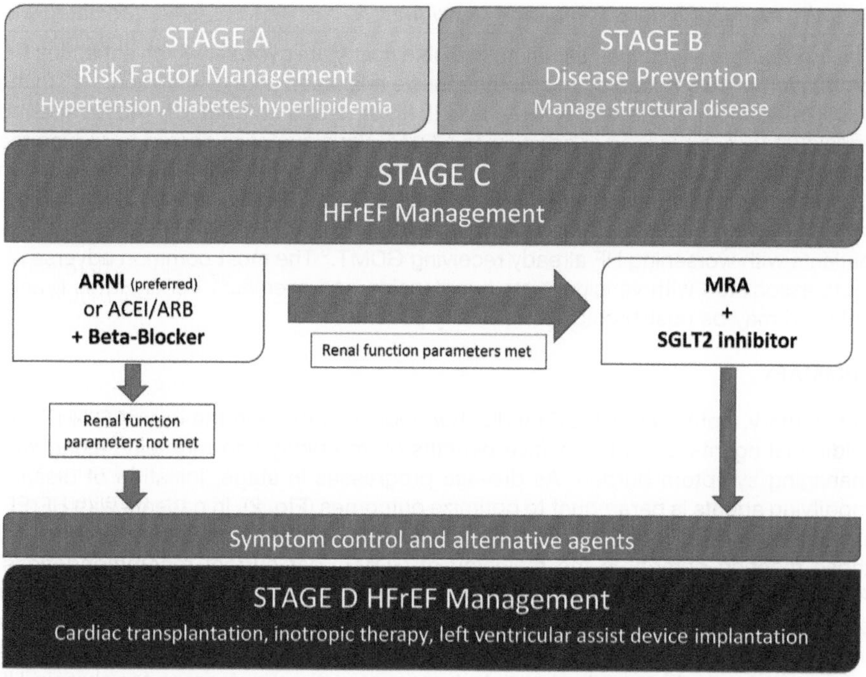

Fig. 2. HFrEF stage progression and management. ACEI, angiotensin converting enzyme inhibitor; ARB, angiotensin receptor blocker; ARNI, angiotensin receptor-neprilysin inhibitor; HFrEF, heart failure with reduced ejection fraction; MRA, mineralocorticoid receptor antagonist; SGLT2, sodium-glucose cotransporter.

a BB, were randomized to receive ivabradine versus placebo. There was a statistically significant reduction in the primary composite outcome of CV death or hospitalization due to worsening HF which was primarily driven by reduction in hospitalizations.[35] Ivabradine is currently recommended for symptomatic patients receiving GDMT (including a BB at the maximum tolerated dose), in sinus rhythm, with a resting HR $\geq$ 70 bpm.[5] Owing to its effects on HR, bradycardia is commonly associated with ivabradine.[34] Cost considerations should be taken into account before prescribing ivabradine as it is brand-only and more expensive than other additive agents.

Digoxin

Digoxin is a cardiac glycoside that exerts its mechanism of action in HF by inhibiting the sodium–potassium ATPase pump in myocardial tissue. This leads to an increase of sodium intracellularly, leading to an influx of calcium, and thus, the net result in an increase in heart contractility.[36] Currently, there is limited evidence that predates GDMT of the utility of digoxin in managing HF. In studies, digoxin was not shown to reduce mortality, but moderately decreased the composite outcome of death and HF hospitalization. Later retrospective data supported its reduction in hospitalizations due to HF. Digoxin requires close monitoring of serum levels as elevated concentrations have been associated with detrimental outcomes, including death. The goal serum concentrations of digoxin in HF is 0.5 to 0.9 ng/mL. GDMT should be optimized before addition of digoxin to HF regimens.[5] Side effects of digoxin include gastrointestinal upset, visual disturbances, and lethargy.[36]

Soluble Guanylyl Cyclase Stimulator, Vericiguat

The novel agent, vericiguat, stimulates soluble guanylate cyclase, which enhances the production of cGMP leading to smooth muscle relaxation and vasodilation.[37,38] In the VICTORIA trial, patients with NYHA class II, III, or IV and an LVEF of $\leq$45% received vericiguat versus placebo in addition to GDMT. Vericiguat was shown to reduce the composite outcome of CV death or HF hospitalization in patients hospitalized within the last 6 months or those that received intravenous diuretic therapy without hospitalization. Current guidelines recommend consideration of the agent in select high-risk patients with worsening HF already receiving GDMT.[5] The most common adverse effects associated with vericiguat are hypotension and anemia.[37] Vericiguat is brand-only and may be cost-prohibitive for many patients.

SUMMARY

In summary, optimizing HFrEF medication regimens through the use of GDMT and additional agents leads to positive benefits on morbidity and mortality, along with managing symptom burden. As disease progresses in stage, initiation of disease modifying agents is paramount to optimize outcomes (**Fig. 2**). In patients with HFrEF, the use of an ARNI (or ACEI/ARB) in addition to a BB, MRA, and SGLT2 inhibitor (for those meeting criteria) is the mainstay of GDMT, per current recommendations. Addition of agents, such as loop diuretics for fluid retention and vasodilators for select patients, has further improved outcomes in patients with HFrEF. With the increasing public health burden of this disease, careful consideration should be taken when selecting medical agents to ensure optimal outcomes for chronic HF patients.

CLINICS CARE POINTS

- Heart failure with reduced ejection fraction (HFrEF) is a chronic disease carrying a significant public health burden.
- Despite long-standing availability of life-saving and morbidity limiting treatment options, there remains a consistent underutilization of guideline-directed medical therapy (GDMT).
- All patients with a diagnosis of HFrEF should be initiated on an angiotensin II receptor blocker with neprilysin inhibitor (preferred), angiotensin-converting enzyme inhibitor, or angiotensin receptor blocker, plus an evidence-based beta-blocker, titrated to target or maximum tolerated doses.
- Patients should be assessed for addition of other appropriate GDMT, with choice of agents driven by patient-specific factors, including comorbidities, adherence and financial considerations.

DISCLOSURE

The authors have nothing to disclose.

REFERENCES

1. Virani SS, Alonso A, Benjamin EJ, et al. Heart disease and stroke statistics—2020 update: a report from the American Heart Association. Circulation 2020;141(9).
2. Centers for Disease Control and Prevention. Heart Failure. Available at: https://www.cdc.gov/heartdisease/heart_failure.htm. Accessed on June 22, 2022.

3. Gerber Y, Weston SA, Redfield MM, et al. A contemporary appraisal of the heart failure epidemic in Olmsted County, Minnesota, 2000 to 2010. JAMA Intern Med 2015;175(6):996.
4. Greene Stephen J, Butler Javed, Albert Nancy M, et al. Medical therapy for heart failure with reduced ejection fraction. J Am Coll Card 2018;72(4):351–66.
5. Heidenreich PA, Bozkurt B, Aguilar D, et al. 2022 aha/acc/hfsa guideline for the management of heart failure: a report of the american college of cardiology/american heart association joint committee on clinical practice guidelines. Circulation. 2022 0(0):10.1161/CIR.0000000000001063.
6. Maddox Thomas M, Januzzi James L, Allen Larry A, et al. 2021 update to the 2017 acc expert consensus decision pathway for optimization of heart failure treatment: answers to 10 pivotal issues about heart failure with reduced ejection fraction. J Am Coll Card 2021;77(6):772–810.
7. Sacubitril and valsartan. Lexi-Drugs. Hudson, OH: Lexicomp. 2022. Available at: http://online.lexi.com/. Updated April 19, 2022. [Accessed 22 April 2022].
8. McMurrary JJV, Packer M, Desae AS, et al. Angiotensin-neprilysin inhibition versus enalapril in heart failure. N Engl J Med 2014;371(11):993–1004.
9. Januzzi JL, Prescott MF, Butler J, et al. Association of change in n-terminal pro–b-type natriuretic peptide following initiation of sacubitril-valsartan treatment with cardiac structure and function in patients with heart failure with reduced ejection fraction. J Am Med Assoc 2019;322(11):1085.
10. Lexi-Drugs Lisinopril, Hudson OH. Lexicomp. 2022. Available at: http://online.lexi.com/. Updated April 30, 2022. [Accessed 30 April 2022].
11. Yancy CW, Jessup M, Bozkurt B, et al. ACC/AHA/HFSA focused update of the 2013 AACR/AHA guideline for the management of heart failure: a report of the American College of Cardiology/American Heart Association task force on clinical practice guidelines and the Heart Failure Society of America. Circulation 2017;136(6).
12. Bratsos S. Efficacy of angiotensin converting enzyme inhibitors and angiotensin receptor-neprilysin inhibitors in the treatment of chronic heart failure: a review of landmark trials. Cureus 2019;11(1):e3913.
13. Effects of enalapril on mortality in severe congestive heart failure. N Engl J Med 1987;316(23):1429–35.
14. Effect of enalapril on survival in patients with reduced left ventricular ejection fractions and congestive heart failure. N Engl J Med 1991;325(5):293–302.
15. Young JB, Dunlap ME, Pfeffer MA, et al. Mortality and morbidity reduction with candesartan in patients with chronic heart failure and left ventricular systolic dysfunction. Circulation 2004;110(17):2618–26.
16. Pitt B, Poole-Wilson PA, Segal R, et al. Effect of losartan compared with captopril on mortality in patients with symptomatic heart failure: randomised trial–the Losartan Heart Failure Survival Study ELITE II. Lancet 2000;355(9215):1582–7.
17. Carvedilol. Lexi-Drugs. Hudson, OH: Lexicomp. 2022. Available at: http://online.lexi.com/. Updated April 21, 2022. [Accessed 22 April 2022].
18. Foody JM, Farrell MH, Krumholz HM. B-blocker therapy in heart failure: scientific review. J Am Med Assoc 2002;287(7):883.
19. Gheorghiade M, Colucci WS, Swedberg K. B-blockers in chronic heart failure. Circulation 2003;107(12):1570–5.
20. CIBIS-II Writers. The Cardiac Insufficiency Bisoprolol Study II (CIBIS-II): a randomised trial. Lancet 1999;353(9146):9–13.
21. Hjalmarson Å, Goldstein S, Fagerberg B, et al. Effects of controlled-release metoprolol on total mortality, hospitalizations, and well-being in patients with heart

failure: the metoprolol cr/xl randomized intervention trial in congestive heart failure(Merit-hf). J Am Med Assoc 2000;283(10):1295.
22. Eichhorn EJ, Bristow MR. The carvedilol prospective randomized cumulative survival (Copernicus) trial. Curr Control Trials Cardiovasc Med 2001;2(1):20–3.
23. Spironolactone. Lexi-Drugs. Hudson, OH: Lexicomp. 2022. Available at: http://online.lexi.com/. Updated April 19, 2022. [Accessed 25 April 2022].
24. Pitt B, Zannad F, Remme WJ, et al. The effect of spironolactone on morbidity and mortality in patients with severe heart failure. N Engl J Med 1999;341(10):709–17.
25. Zannad F, McMurray JJV, Krum H, et al. Eplerenone in patients with systolic heart failure and mild symptoms. N Engl J Med 2011;364(1):11–21.
26. MCMurray JJV, Solomon SD, Inzucchi SE, et al. Dapagliflozin in patients with heart failure with reduced ejection fraction. N Engl J Med 2019;381:1995–2008.
27. Packer M, Anker AD, Butler J, et al. Cardiovascular and renal outcomes with empagliflozin in heart failure. N Engl J Med 2020;383:1413–24.
28. Lam CSP, Chandramouli C, Ahooja V, et al. SGLT2 inhibitors in heart failure: current management, unmet needs, and therapeutic prospects. J Am Heart Assoc 2019;8:e013389.
29. Dapagliflozin. Lexi-Drug. Hudson, OH: Lexicomp. 2022. Available at: http://online.lexi.com/. Updated April 19, 2022. [Accessed 30 April 2022].
30. Empagliflozin. Lexi-Drug. Hudson, OH: Lexicomp. 2022. Available at: http://online.lexi.com/. Updated April 19, 2022. [Accessed 30 April 2022].
31. Cohn JN, Archibald DG, Ziesche S, et al. Effect of vasodilatory therapy on mortality in chronic congestive heart failure. N Engl J Med 1986;314:1584.
32. Taylor AL, Ziesche S, Yancy C, et al. Combination of isosorbide dinitrate and hydralazine in blacks with heart failure. N Engl J Med 2004;351:2049–57.
33. Furosemide. Lexi-Drug. Hudson, OH: Lexicomp. 2022. Available at: http://online.lexi.com/. Updated March 28, 2022. [Accessed 30 April 2022].
34. Ivabradine. Lexi-Drug. Hudson, OH: Lexicomp. 2022. Available at: http://online.lexi.com/. Updated April 19, 2022. [Accessed 30 April 2022].
35. Swedberg K, Komajda M, Bohm M, et al. Ivabradine and outcomes in chronic heart failure: a randomised placebo-controlled study. Lancet 2010;376:875–85.
36. Digoxin. Lexi-Drug. Hudson, OH: Lexicomp. 2022. Available at: http://online.lexi.com/. Updated April 19, 2022. [Accessed 30 April 2022].
37. Vericiguat [package insert]. Whitehouse Station, NJ: Merck & Co., Inc.. Available at: https://www.accessdata.fda.gov/drugsatfda_docs/label/2021/214377s000lbl.pdf. Accesed June 22, 2022.
38. Armstrong PW, Pieske B, Anstrom KJ, et al. Vericiguat in patients with heart failure and reduced ejection fraction. N Engl J Med 2020;382:1883–93.

Medications When the Brain Is Hurt

Jessica Starr, PharmD, BCPS[a,*], Victoria Trott, PA-C, MMS[b]

KEYWORDS

- Ischemic stroke • Intracerebral hemorrhage • Stroke • Tissue plasminogen activator • Antiplatelet therapy

KEY POINTS

- Stroke is the second leading cause of disability and death worldwide.
- Early detection of ischemic or hemorrhagic stroke is critical for early intervention and improved outcomes for patients.
- Management of modifiable risk factors can significantly reduce the risk of ischemic and hemorrhagic stroke.
- Initiating early interventions for acute stroke can reduce ischemia and improve the outcomes of patients.

INTRODUCTION

Every 40 seconds someone in the United States has a stroke.[1] The impact of stroke on an individual's physical and emotional state can be lifechanging. As a physician assistant (PA), identifying and appropriately managing patients with modifiable risk factors and nonmodifiable risk factors is an important step to assist in reducing the risk of stroke. As a PA, quickly detecting the signs and symptoms will allow for rapid intervention and ultimately provide the best possible outcome for patients. In a matter of minutes, you can make a significant difference in a patient's life.

Epidemiology

Stroke is the second leading cause of disability and death worldwide.[2] There are 795,000 new or recurrent strokes each year with 610,000 being first attacks and 185,000 recurrent attacks.[1] Ischemic stroke accounts for approximately 87% of all strokes. Ischemic stroke can further be divided into lacunar (23%) or non-lacunar stroke (77%).[3] A transient ischemic attack (TIA) is a transient episode of neurologic dysfunction and significantly increases the risk of a subsequent ischemic stroke.[4] The incidence of TIA is 1.19/1000 person-years.[5] Hemorrhagic stroke, which accounts

[a] Auburn University Harrison School of Pharmacy, 2316 Walker Building, Auburn, AL 36849, USA; [b] Annapolis Neurology Associates, 122 Defense Highway, Suite 210, Annapolis, MD 21401, USA
* Correspondent author.
E-mail address: jas0003@auburn.edu

Physician Assist Clin 8 (2023) 259–268
https://doi.org/10.1016/j.cpha.2022.10.006

for the remaining 13% of strokes, is divided into intracerebral hemorrhage (ICH) and subarachnoid hemorrhage.[1]

Etiology

Ischemic stroke is an acute onset of focal neurologic deficit that involves permanent infarction of central nervous system tissue. This is caused by an occlusion within a cerebral artery (thrombotic stroke) or an embolus originating in the carotid arteries or the ventricles of the heart (embolic stroke). Atherosclerosis of the carotid arteries leads to plaque formation and if plaque ruptures, collagen is exposed resulting in platelet aggregation and thrombus formation. The clot may break off and cause cranial vessel occlusion resulting in ischemia. Strokes originating from a cardioembolic source are presumed to originate from thrombus formation in the left ventricle. Lacunar strokes are typically caused by small vessel disease.[6] Non-lacunar strokes are cryptogenic (45%) with no confirmed source, cardioembolic (35%), or due to large artery atherosclerosis (17%).[3] A TIA is also caused by an occlusion within a cerebral artery or embolus originating in the carotid arteries or the ventricles of the heart. However, it differs from an ischemic stroke in that it is caused by focal brain, spinal cord, or retinal ischemia, without acute infarction.[4]

An ICH is caused by a rupture of a small artery generally secondary to hypertensive changes or other vascular abnormalities.[7] A subarachnoid hemorrhage occurs when there is bleeding between the brain and subarachnoid space. The most common causes are head trauma or ruptured brain aneurysm.

Risk Factors

Risk factors for ischemic stroke can be described as nonmodifiable or modifiable (**Table 1**).[1]

Although many of the risk factors for ICH are the same as ischemic stroke, the most significant is hypertension. Other risks for ICH include old age, excessive alcohol use, current smoker, Asian ethnicity, illicit drug use, hypocholesterolemia, and male sex. Encouraging patients to control modifiable risk factors can reduce the risk of ischemic stroke and ICH.

Clinical Presentation

Clinical presentation of ischemic stroke includes weakness on one side of the body, visual impairment in one or both eyes, confusion, inability to speak or understand speech, sudden and severe headache with no known cause, facial drooping, numbness on one side of the body, vertigo, and loss of balance and falling. The specific areas of neurologic deficit are determined by the area of the brain involved.[6] The National Institutes of Health Stroke Scale (NIHSS) is commonly used to assess the severity of stroke based on a patient's signs and symptoms. Scores range from 0 to 42 with higher scores indicating greater severity.[9] Key laboratory tests in acute ischemic stroke include an assessment of coagulation parameters (INR, aPTT), platelet count, and blood glucose.[9] Diagnosis is confirmed via computed tomography (CT) scanning and/or MRI. CT scans should reveal an area of hypointensity, but it may take 24 hours before the scan shows an infarction. The MRI can reveal areas of ischemia with higher resolution and diffusion-weighed imaging. The MRI can reveal an infarct within minutes of stroke onset. Carotid Dopplers can be used to determine extracranial carotid artery stenosis. An electrocardiogram (ECG) can help rule in or rule out atrial fibrillation. Vascular imaging with computed tomography angiography should be done in patients being considered for endovascular treatment.[9]

Table 1
Risk factors for ischemic stroke[1]

Nonmodifiable	
Age	Increased risk in patients > or = to 65 y of age. Incidence of stroke doubles every 10 y after age 55
Low birth weight	Increased mortality rate in patients with low birth weight
Race/ethnicity	Increased risk in African American and Hispanic/Latino American populations
Genetics	Increased risk with positive family history
Gender	Men have a greater risk than women
Modifiable	
Hypertension	Increased risk with blood pressure >130/80 mm Hg
Dyslipidemia	Increased risk when LDL cholesterol (LDL-C) is > 100 mg/dL
Diabetes	Increased risk of 1.5 times in diabetics vs nondiabetics
Cigarette smoking	Increased risk by 12% for each increment of five cigarettes per day[8]

Prevention

Primary prevention against ischemic stroke focuses on the reduction of modifiable risk factors (see **Table 1**).[10] Hypertension is the most important modifiable risk factor. The target blood pressure is < 130/80 mm Hg.[10] Medications, dietary changes, and exercise are the primary ways to achieve this goal. Reducing sodium intake, limiting alcohol consumption, increasing potassium intake, and following a diet, such as the dietary approaches to stop hypertension (DASH) diet, are the recommended dietary changes for hypertension.[11] The American College of Sports Medicine (ACSM) recommends moderate intensity, aerobic exercise 5 to 7 days per week, as well as resistance exercise 2 to 3 days per week and flexibility exercise > or = 2 to 3 days per week.[12] These recommendations are also in line with the American College of Cardiology and American Heart Association.[10]

Controlling dyslipidemia with the use of statin therapy in addition to lifestyle modifications decrease the risk of stroke in high-risk patients (ie, coronary artery disease or diabetes).[10] ACSM recommends moderate-to-vigorous intensity aerobic exercise 30 to 60 minutes per day and up to 50 to 60 minutes per day to assist with weight loss, as well as a resistance exercise for individuals with dyslipidemia.[13] In addition, dietary changes include reducing intake of saturated and *trans* fats, increasing polyunsaturated and monounsaturated fats, adding tree nuts to the diet, fortifying foods with plant stanols and sterols, reducing alcohol consumption to one to two drinks per day and following a diet, such as the Mediterranean diet.[10]

Optimizing blood glucose levels can help reduce the risk of damage to blood vessels. The goal is to reduce blood glucose levels to <140 mg/dL. Reducing blood glucose levels is accomplished with the use of medication, dietary changes (ie, DASH diet), and 150 minutes of moderate-intensity exercise per week.[14]

Smoking cessation among current smokers and abstaining from cigarette smoking by nonsmokers decreases the risk of stroke. If needed, medications and nicotine replacement therapy can assist current smokers in cessation.[10]

Treatment of Ischemic Stroke

The immediate goal of therapy in ischemic stroke is to reduce neurologic injury and long-term disability. Once the patient is through the hyperacute period, the goal of therapy is to prevent reoccurrence and decrease mortality.

Acute Treatment of Ischemic Stroke

The treatment of acute ischemic stroke has a narrow therapeutic window; therefore, a timely evaluation and diagnosis are essential. Pharmacologic agents recommended by the American Heart Association Stroke Council for acute stroke treatment are recombinant tissue plasminogen activator (rtPA/Activase), aspirin, and the combination of aspirin plus clopidogrel.[9]

Tissue Plasminogen Activator

rtPA is a fibrinolytic agent able to achieve early reperfusion and improve neurologic outcomes.[15] rtPA exerts its effects via the initiation of local fibrinolysis. It binds directly to fibrin thereby causing plasminogen to convert to plasmin. Plasmin is the enzyme responsible for clot dissolution. rtPA is administered intravenously at a dose of 0.9 mg/kg with a maximum dose of 90 mg in patients weighing >100 kg. rtPA should be administered within 4.5 hours of symptom onset; however, the ideal window of opportunity is 60 minutes.[9] If the time of onset is unknown, patients are ineligible to receive rtPA. Due to its effects on fibrin, rtPA puts patients at risk for major bleeding. The American Heart Association Stroke Council details extensive exclusion criteria (**Box 1**).[9,15] There are also several relative exclusions for which the benefits and risks of giving rtPA must be carefully weighed. Some of these relative exclusions are pregnancy, recent major surgery, and recent acute myocardial infarction (see **Box 1**).

Aspirin

Aspirin decreases morbidity and mortality when administered within 24 to 48 hours of stroke onset.[9] The recommended initial dose is 160 to 325 mg. Aspirin does not alter the neurologic outcomes of stroke; aspirin prevents recurrent strokes. If a patient receives rtPA, aspirin and other antithrombotic agents should be held for at least 24 hours after rtPA is administered.[9]

Aspirin + clopidogrel

The combination of aspirin plus clopidogrel should only be initiated in patients who present with a minor ischemic stroke (NIHSS $\leq$ 3) or TIA.[3,9] This combination should only be given to patients who did not receive rtPA if it can be initiated within 24 hours of symptom onset and should only be continued for 21 to 90 days.

HYPERTENSION

Most patients present with elevated or normal blood pressure. Neurologic deterioration occurs with low and high blood pressures. Blood pressure treatment should be withheld unless systolic blood pressure is above 220 mm Hg or diastolic blood pressure is above 120 mm Hg.[9] However, if a patient meets all other criteria for rtPA, except elevated blood pressure, the recommendation is to decrease the blood pressure to <185/110 mm Hg before rtPA administration.[9] Frequent blood pressure monitoring should occur during rtPA administration and the subsequent 24 hours. Several antihypertensive agents are recommended for use during acute stroke. These include labetalol, nicardipine, and sodium nitroprusside (**Table 2**).[9] Sodium nitroprusside is reserved for blood pressure not controlled by labetalol and nicardipine, and it should be used with caution in patients with renal insufficiency because of the risk of cyanide toxicity with prolonged use. If antihypertensive therapy is necessary, the blood pressure should be decreased by approximately 15% within the first day.

Box 1
Exclusion criteria for recombinant tissue plasminogen activator[9,15]

- Symptom onset >4.5 h
- Mild nondisabling stroke (NIHSS score 0–5)
- Current intracranial hemorrhage
- Severe head trauma, prior ischemic stroke, or intracranial/spinal surgery in the previous 3 months
- History of intracranial or subarachnoid hemorrhage
- Gastrointestinal (GI) malignancy or GI bleeding within the previous 21 days
- CT with extensive regions of hypoattenuation
- Platelets <100,000 mm^3, INR >1.7, aPTT >40s or PT > 15 s
- Full treatment dose of low-molecular-weight heparin (LMWH) within the previous 24 hours
- Current use of direct thrombin inhibitors or direct factor Xa inhibitors with elevated sensitivity lab tests or previous dose within 48 hours
- Sustained elevated blood pressure (systolic >185 or diastolic > 110 mm Hg)
- Sustained blood glucose <50 mg/dL
- Concomitant abciximab therapy
- Concomitant infective endocarditis
- Concomitant aortic arch dissection
- Intra-axial intracranial neoplasm

Secondary Prevention of Ischemic Stroke

Patients with a history of an ischemic stroke have a significantly increased risk of having another stroke.[3] The American Heart Association Stroke Council recommends several different pharmacotherapy options for secondary prevention.

Antiplatelet Therapy

The mainstay of therapy is long-term treatment with an antiplatelet agent; however, lowering blood pressure and cholesterol is also important. Currently, aspirin, clopidogrel, and extended-release dipyridamole plus aspirin are all acceptable antiplatelet options for initial therapy.[3] The American Heart Association Stroke Council does not give preference for one agent over another (**Table 3**). Ticlopidine is not recommended for use. Patients with a TIA or acute minor stroke may benefit from dual antiplatelet therapy with aspirin and clopidogrel for 21 to 90 days. For patients already taking aspirin at the time of stroke, the effectiveness of increasing the dose of aspirin or changing to another antiplatelet medication is not well established.

Aspirin is the most well-studied antiplatelet agent used in the secondary prevention of stroke. Aspirin's antithrombotic effects occur by irreversible inhibition of platelet cyclooxygenase ultimately leading to a reduction in platelet aggregation.[16] The current dosing recommendation varies from 50 to 325 mg/d[3] Most studies have shown that low- and high-dose aspirin prevent the reoccurrence of stroke. However, higher doses of aspirin are associated with a greater risk of gastrointestinal hemorrhage. Adverse reactions include gastritis, gastrointestinal ulcerations, and duodenal ulcers.

Clopidogrel works through selective, irreversible inhibition of adenosine diphosphate-induced platelet aggregation.[17] It is given as a 75-mg tablet once daily.[3]

Table 2
Medications for acute blood pressure lowering[9]

Medication	Onset (min)	Duration (min)	Dose
Labetalol	5–10	180–360	10–20 mg IV bolus x 1, can repeat x 1 OR start 2 mg/h
Nicardipine	5–10	15–30	5 mg/h, titrate every 5–15 min to max of 15 mg/h
Sodium nitroprusside	Immediate	1–2	0.3–0.5 mcg/kg/min titrated every few min Max of 10 mcg/kg/min

The safety of clopidogrel is comparable to aspirin and the incidence of neutropenia and thrombotic thrombocytopenic purpura is low. Clopidogrel is an alternative to aspirin in those patients who are allergic to aspirin. The combination of clopidogrel with aspirin is not recommended for long-term secondary prevention as there is an increased risk of hemorrhage.[3]

Dipyridamole inhibits phosphodiesterase resulting in the accumulation of adenosine and cyclic-3′,5′-adenosine monophosphate, and platelet aggregation inhibition.[18] The combination of aspirin and dipyridamole is given as a capsule that contains dipyridamole extended-release pellets in 200 mg and immediate-release aspirin in 25 mg.[3] The combination capsule is taken twice daily. The adverse effects include headache, dyspepsia, and abdominal pain.

Ticlopidine is not recommended by the American Heart Association Stroke Council because of side effects.[3] Ticlopidine causes severe gastrointestinal effects, neutropenia, agranulocytosis, aplastic anemia, and thrombotic thrombocytopenic purpura.[19]

Hypertension

Antihypertensive treatment is recommended for patients with a history of ischemic stroke who are beyond the first 48 hours, regardless of the patient's prior medical history.[3,20] The target blood pressure is < 130/80 mm Hg. Data support a thiazide-type diuretic, angiotensin-converting enzyme (ACE) inhibitors, or angiotensin II receptor blocker (ARBs).[3] Thiazide-type diuretics, such as hydrochlorothiazide, inhibit the reabsorption of sodium in the distal convoluted tubules in the kidney.[21] This causes an increased excretion of both sodium and water, which leads to a reduction in blood pressure. ACE inhibitors, such as lisinopril, are competitive inhibitors of ACE which prevents the conversion of angiotensin I to angiotensin II, thereby, causing

Table 3
Antiplatelet therapy recommendations for the secondary prevention of ischemic stroke[3]

Antiplatelet Therapy	Recommendation
Aspirin 50–325 mg po daily Clopidogrel 75 mg po daily Extended-release dipyridamole 200 mg plus aspirin 25 mg po twice daily	Acceptable initial therapy
Aspirin + clopidogrel	For recent minor (NIHSS score ≤3) ischemic stroke or high-risk TIA if initiated early (within 12–24 h of symptom onset and at least within 7 d) and continued for only 21–90 d, followed by monotherapy

Table 4
Statin therapy

Statin	Renal Considerations	Select Drug Interactions
Atorvastatin	No dose adjustment	Metabolized by CYP3A. Some medications that significantly inhibit its metabolism include erythromycin, clarithromycin, ketoconazole, verapamil, nefazodone, protease inhibitors, cyclosporine, and grapefruit juice.
Fluvastatin	Use with caution in severe impairment, particularly doses daily doses over 40 mg	Metabolized by CYP2C9. Less likely to be involved in drug interactions.
Lovastatin	If CrCl <30 mL/min, use with caution, particularly doses over 20 mg	Metabolized by CYP3A. Some medications that significantly inhibit its metabolism include erythromycin, clarithromycin, ketoconazole, verapamil, nefazodone, protease inhibitors, cyclosporine, and grapefruit juice.
Pravastatin	In severe renal impairment, start with 10 mg daily	Not significantly metabolized by cytochrome P450 and may be less likely to be involved in drug interactions.
Simvastatin	No dose adjustment	Metabolized by CYP3A. Some medications that significantly inhibit its metabolism include erythromycin, clarithromycin, ketoconazole, verapamil, nefazodone, protease inhibitors, cyclosporine, and grapefruit juice. Do not exceed 20 mg daily with amiodarone or verapamil.

vasodilation.[22] ARBs, such as losartan, antagonize the receptor site of angiotensin II, thereby, preventing angiotensin II from binding, which causes vasodilation.[23]

Hyperlipidemia

Patients with atherosclerotic ischemic stroke should receive HMG-CoA reductase inhibitors (statins) with intensive lipid-lowering effects to reduce the risk of recurrent events.[3,24] High-intensity statin therapy should be indicated in all patients. Statins, such as atorvastatin, are selective, competitive inhibitors of HMG-CoA reductase, which is the enzyme responsible for converting HMG-CoA to mevalonate. Reducing the synthesis of cholesterol leads to an upregulation of LDL receptors and an increase in the hepatic uptake of LDL. If the LDL-C remains > 70 mg/dL, ezetimibe can be added to reduce the risk of events (**Table 4**).[3,24] Ezetimibe inhibits the absorption of cholesterol in the small intestines, thereby, reducing blood cholesterol.[25]

Treatment of Intracerebral Hemorrhage

The management of ICH depends on its etiology and severity. However, early intervention is critical. These interventions first begin with basic life support, and then, initiating medications to control seizures, blood pressure, intracranial pressure, and bleeding.[26]

Box 2
2015 AHA/ASA guidelines for blood pressure control in ICH[26]

If the systolic blood pressure (SBP) is between 150 and 200 mm Hg, lower the SBP to 140 mm Hg.

If the SBP is > 220 mm Hf, it may be reasonable to consider an aggressive reduction of BP with a continuous intravenous infusion and frequent monitoring.

The frequency of clinical seizure activity can be as high as 16% among patients suffering from ICH with the highest incidence occurring within the first week.[16] In many cases, these seizures are nonconvulsive. The American Heart Association/American Stroke Association (AHA/ASA) advises antiepileptic therapy for patients with clinical seizure activity, or for patients with a change in mental status who have electroencephalographic (EEG) seizure activity. Early intervention with benzodiazepines, such as lorazepam or diazepam, is recommended. For prolonged control, adding phenytoin or fosphenytoin may be necessary. However, prophylactic anti-seizure medications are not recommended.[26]

Patients with ICH often present with elevated blood pressure. Although current evidence is limited, early and intensive blood pressure lowering is safe in patients with ICH and shows a favorable trend in the reduction of death and major disability.[26] The 2015 AHA/ASA guidelines for blood pressure control are given in **Box 2.**[26]

Increased intracranial pressure can occur from surrounding edema, the hematoma, or both. Recommendations for initial management include elevating the bed 30°, keeping the head midline, analgesics, sedatives, and antacids. Alternative therapies include osmotic agents, such as mannitol and hypertonic saline.[26]

SUMMARY

If you have known a patient, friend, or family member who has suffered from a stroke, you have seen within a matter of seconds, minutes, or hours the significant impact it can have on their lives. Not only can stroke cause lifelong disability for patients, but it also changes the lives of those around them. Therefore, both patients and providers must work together to reduce modifiable risk factors through lifestyle modifications and medication management. Early identification, an appropriate history, physical examination, and brain imaging allow for rapid intervention and reduce the long-term effects of an acute stroke.

CLINICS CARE POINTS

Pearls

- Lifestyle modifications and medication management can reduce modifiable risk factors and ultimately the risk of stroke
- Advanced imaging tools are available to detect ischemic and ICH
- After a stroke has occurred, initiating secondary prevention can reduce the risk of recurrent stroke

Pitfalls

- Inability to reduce modifiable risk factors will lead to a higher risk of stroke
- Without early detection and intervention, both ischemic and ICH can lead to lifelong disability
- Without early detection, tPA cannot be initiated after 4.5 hours for ischemic stroke

DISCLOSURE

The authors have no conflicts to disclose.

REFERENCES

1. Tsao CW, Aday AW, Almarzooq ZI, et al. Heart disease and stroke statistics-2022 update: a report from the american heart association. Circulation 2022;145(8): e153–639. https://doi.org/10.1161/CIR.0000000000000105.
2. Saini V, Guada L, Yavagal DR. Global epidemiology of stroke and access to acute ischemic stroke interventions. Neurology 2021;97(20 Suppl 2):S6–16. https://doi.org/10.1212/WNL.0000000000012781.
3. Kleindorfer DO, Towfighi A, Chaturvedi S, et al. 2021 guideline for the prevention of stroke in patients with stroke and transient ischemic attack: a guideline from the american heart association/american stroke association. Stroke 2021;52(7): e364–e*467* [published correction appears in Stroke. 2021 Jul;52(7):e483-e484].
4. Easton JD, Saver JL, Albers GW, et al. Definition and evaluation of transient ischemic attack: a scientific statement for healthcare professionals from the American Heart Association/American Stroke Association Stroke Council; Council on Cardiovascular Surgery and Anesthesia; Council on Cardiovascular Radiology and Intervention; Council on Cardiovascular Nursing; and the Interdisciplinary Council on Peripheral Vascular Disease. The American Academy of Neurology affirms the value of this statement as an educational tool for neurologists. Stroke 2009;40(6):2276–93. https://doi.org/10.1161/STROKEAHA.108.192218.
5. Lioutas VA, Ivan CS, Himali JJ, et al. Incidence of Transient Ischemic Attack and Association With Long-term Risk of Stroke. JAMA 2021;325(4):373–81. https://doi.org/10.1001/jama.2020.25071.
6. Smith WS, Johnston S, Hemphill J III. Ischemic Stroke. In: Jameson J, Fauci AS, Kasper DL, et al, editors. Harrison's Principles of Internal Medicine, 20e. McGraw Hill; 2018. Available at: https://accesspharmacy.mhmedical.com/content.aspx?bookid=2129&sectionid=192532037. Accessed March 10, 2022.
7. An SJ, Kim TJ, Yoon BW. Epidemiology, Risk Factors, and Clinical Features of Intracerebral Hemorrhage: An Update. J Stroke 2017;19(1):3–10. https://doi.org/10.5853/jos.2016.00864.
8. Pan B, Jin X, Jun L, et al. The relationship between smoking and stroke: A meta-analysis. Medicine (Baltimore) 2019;98(12):e14872. https://doi.org/10.1097/MD.0000000000014872.
9. Powers WJ, Rabinstein AA, Ackerson T, et al. Guidelines for the Early Management of Patients With Acute Ischemic Stroke: 2019 Update to the 2018 Guidelines for the Early Management of Acute Ischemic Stroke: A Guideline for Healthcare Professionals From the American Heart Association/American Stroke Association. Stroke 2019;50(12):e344–418. https://doi.org/10.1161/STR.0000000000000211 [published correction appears in Stroke. 2019 Dec;50(12):e440-e441].
10. Arnett DK, Blumenthal RS, Albert MA, et al. 2019 ACC/AHA Guideline on the Primary Prevention of Cardiovascular Disease: A Report of the American College of Cardiology/American Heart Association Task Force on Clinical Practice Guidelines. Circulation 2019;140(11):e596–646 [published correction appears in Circulation. 2019;140(11):e649-e650] [published correction appears in Circulation. 2020 Jan 28;141(4):e60] [published correction appears in Circulation. 2020 Apr 21;141(16):e774].
11. Bazzano LA, Green T, Harrison TN, et al. Dietary approaches to prevent hypertension. Curr Hypertens Rep 2013;15(6):694–702.

12. ACSM_CMS. ACSM Blog. [online]. 2022. Available at: https://www.acsm.org/blog-detail/acsm-certified-blog/2019/02/27/exercise-hypertension-prevention-treatment. Accessed 30 January 2022.
13. Professional.heart.org. 2022. Physical Activity as a Critical Component of First-Line Treatment of Elevated Blood Pressure or Cholesterol: Who, What, and How?. Available at: https://professional.heart.org/en/science-news/physical-activity-as-a-critical-component-of-first-line treatment-for-elevated-bp-or cholesterol/Commentary#:~:text=Accordingly%2C%20ACSM%20recommends%20adults%20with,impact%20resistance%20exercise%20has%20on. Accessed 30 January 2022.
14. gov Cdc. Get Active! | Diabetes | CDC. [online]. 2022. Available at: https://www.cdc.gov/diabetes/managing/active.html. Accessed 30 January 2022.
15. Genentech, Inc. Activase [package insert]. U.S. Food and Drug Administration website. Available at: https://www.accessdata.fda.gov/drugsatfda_docs/label/2015/103172s5203lbl.pdf. Revised February 2015. Accessed March 10, 2022.
16. Aspirin. Lexi-Drugs. Lexicomp. Wolters Kluwer Health, Inc. Riverwoods, IL. Available at: http://online.lexi.com. Accessed March 10, 2022.
17. Clopidogrel. Lexi-Drugs. Lexicomp. Wolters Kluwer Health, Inc. Riverwoods, IL. Available at: http://online.lexi.com. Accessed March 10, 2022.
18. Dipyridamole. Lexi-Drugs. Lexicomp. Wolters Kluwer Health, Inc. Riverwoods, IL. Available at: http://online.lexi.com. Accessed March 10, 2022.
19. Ticlopidine. Lexi-Drugs. Lexicomp. Wolters Kluwer Health, Inc. Riverwoods, IL. Available at: http://online.lexi.com. Accessed March 10, 2022.
20. Whelton PK, Carey RM, Aronow WS, et al. 2017 ACC/AHA/AAPA/ABC/ACPM/AGS/APhA/ASH/ASPC/NMA/PCNA Guideline for the Prevention, Detection, Evaluation, and Management of High Blood Pressure in Adults: A Report of the American College of Cardiology/American Heart Association Task Force on Clinical Practice Guidelines. Hypertension 2018;71(6):e13–115 [published correction appears in Hypertension. 2018;71(6):e140-e144].
21. Hydrochlorothiazide. Lexi-Drugs. Lexicomp. Wolters Kluwer Health, Inc. Riverwoods, IL. Available at: http://online.lexi.com. Accessed March 10, 2022.
22. Lisinopril. Lexi-Drugs. Lexicomp. Wolters Kluwer Health, Inc. Riverwoods, IL. Available at: http://online.lexi.com. Accessed March 10, 2022.
23. Losartan3. Lexi-Drugs. Lexicomp. Wolters Kluwer Health, Inc. Riverwoods, IL. Available at: http://online.lexi.com. Accessed March 10, 2022.
24. Grundy SM, Stone NJ, Bailey AL, et al. 2018 AHA/ACC/AACVPR/AAPA/ABC/ACPM/ADA/AGS/APhA/ASPC/NLA/PCNA Guideline on the Management of Blood Cholesterol: A Report of the American College of Cardiology/American Heart Association Task Force on Clinical Practice Guidelines. Circulation 2019;139(25):e1082–143. https://doi.org/10.1161/CIR.0000000000000625 [published correction appears in Circulation. 2019 Jun 18;139(25):e1182-e1186].
25. Ezetimibe. Lexi-Drugs. Lexicomp. Wolters Kluwer Health, Inc. Riverwoods, IL. Available at: http://online.lexi.com. Accessed March 10, 2022.
26. Hemphill JC 3rd, Greenberg SM, Anderson CS, et al. Guidelines for the management of spontaneous intracerebral hemorrhage: a guideline for healthcare professionals from the american heart association/american stroke association. Stroke 2015;46(7):2032–60.

Managing Diabetes

Jeanna Sewell, PharmD[a,*], Rebecca Johnson, PA-C[b]

KEYWORDS

• Diabetes • Glucose control • Drug therapy

KEY POINTS

- There have been many advancements in therapy for type 2 diabetes.
- Guidance is available to target therapy at patient-specific factors for best clinical outcomes.
- Through advancements in drug therapy we are able to manage diabetes, comorbidities, and diabetes complications.

INTRODUCTION

Clinicians are aware of the public health impact of diabetes. Healthy People 2030 has set specific goals related to diabetes management in hopes of seeing a decrease in not only the number of deaths from diabetes but also the number of new cases of diabetes and complications from the disease.[1] These are attainable goals thanks to the many therapeutic options available today.

Although it is one of the most common chronic diseases in the United States,[1] the management of type 2 diabetes mellitus (T2DM) can be intimidating due to changes in therapeutic guidelines and drug therapy options available; this sometimes leads to less aggressive or inadequate management of the disease.

Many of the newer agents on the market have indications for use in addition to improving glycemic control. There are certain comorbidities that can help guide clinical decision making when selecting an initial or additional agent. In this article, innovations in diabetes treatment are discussed including glucagonlike peptide-1 receptor agonists (GLP-1 RAs), dipeptidyl peptidase-4 (DPP-4) inhibitors, sodium glucose cotransporter 2 (SGLT2) inhibitors, and insulins (**Table 1**).

DISCUSSION

Innovations in Diabetes Treatment

Glucagon-like peptide-1 receptor agonists

GLP-1 RAs are one of the newer and more exciting therapies for T2DM currently on the market. GLP-1 RAs work via various mechanisms that have an impact throughout the

[a] Department of Pharmacy Practice, Auburn University Harrison School of Pharmacy, 1330Q Walker Building, Auburn, AL 36849, USA; [b] Mercy Medical Clinic, 1702A Catherine Court, Auburn, AL 36830, USA

* Corresponding author.

E-mail address: Mjc0001@auburn.edu

Physician Assist Clin 8 (2023) 269–279
https://doi.org/10.1016/j.cpha.2022.10.007
2405-7991/23/Published by Elsevier Inc.

body. Their primary mechanism involves the incretin effect by which they increase insulin secretion, decrease glucagon secretion, and slow gastric emptying.[2] Additional actions are evident in the brain where appetite is seen to decrease. These varied effects throughout the body cause a significant decrease in glycated hemoglobin A_{1c} (HbA_{1c}) of 0.8% to 1.6%.[3]

Several GLP-1 RAs are currently on the market; they are administered twice daily, once daily, or once weekly, depending on the drug and formulation used. Apart from semaglutide (Rybelsus), all GLP-1 RAs are administered subcutaneously; this is important when deciding on therapies because some patients will be resistant to injections. Oral semaglutide requires administration 30 minutes before a meal with 4 ounces of water, but other therapies in the class can be administered without relation to meals.[4] All GLP-1 RAs are currently only available in brand formulations, which can be cost inhibitory for many patients.

GLP-1 RAs have several benefits, but there are some side effects and warnings that prescribers should be aware of. The most common side effects of GLP-1 RAs are abdominal pain, nausea, vomiting, and constipation. Nausea and vomiting are common side effects of GLP-1 RAs but can be significantly limited by slowly titrating to maximum doses.[2] Hypoglycemia is listed as a side effect, but primarily occurs in the setting of concomitant insulin or sulfonylurea use. There are some warnings to take into consideration with use of these therapies including thyroid C-cell tumors, personal or family history of medullary thyroid cancer, or multiple endocrine neoplasia syndrome type 2 (MEN2). There is also a risk of pancreatitis with GLP-1 RA use.[2,5]

Dieptidyl peptidase-4 inhibitors

DPP-4 inhibitors have been in use longer than GLP-1 RAs, with the introduction of sitagliptin in 2006. Drugs in this class also work through the incretin effect, similar to GLP-1 RAs. Through their actions, they prevent the breakdown of incretin hormones by the enzyme DPP-4, thereby increasing insulin synthesis and decreasing glucagon secretion from the pancreas.[6] Generally, DPP-4 inhibitors are not associated with significant weight loss, unlike other newer therapies for treatment of T2DM, but they do not result in weight gain. Expected HbA_{1c} reduction with these therapies is 0.6% to 0.8%.[7]

Side effects and contraindications are limited with DPP-4 inhibitors. The most common side effects reported are nasopharyngitis and joint pain. DPP-4 inhibitors should be avoided in combination with GLP-1 RAs due to the similar mechanism of action and limited HbA_{1c} reduction when combined. Their availability as an oral formulation does make them a good option for many patients who are hesitant to use injectable medications.[7]

Sodium glucose cotransporter 2 inhibitors

SGLT2 inhibitors were first introduced to the market in 2013 with a novel mechanism of action in the treatment of T2DM. These therapies work by inhibiting SGLT2 in the proximal renal tubules, which causes a reduction in the reabsorption of filtered glucose from the tubular lumen and lowers the renal threshold for glucose. By reducing filtered glucose reabsorption and lowering the renal threshold for glucose there is an increase in urinary excretion of glucose, thereby reducing plasma glucose concentrations. Through this mechanism, the drugs in this class lower HbA_{1c} by 0.5% to 0.8%.[8]

SGLT2 inhibitors have several side effects to be aware of, with some being common and others being severe, yet uncommon. Genitourinary side effects are some of the more common side effects and are associated with the mechanism of action of SGLT2 inhibitors. Because SGLT2 inhibitors increase urinary excretion of glucose, glucosuria-induced bacterial growth and increased adherence of bacteria to the uroepithelium have been hypothesized as the reasons that these agents further increase the risk of urinary tract infections and yeast infections in both men and women. These events are generally mild in intensity, respond to treatment, and do not lead to discontinuation of therapy.[9]

Blood pressure reduction can be noted with SGLT2 inhibitor use related to volume loss. Owing to this, some patients may experience hypotension and potentially acute kidney injury. Rare but serious side effects of SGLT2 inhibitors include necrotizing fasciitis of the perineum, also known as Fournier gangrene, increased risk of fracture, and lower limb amputation (primarily seen with canagliflozin). Diabetic ketoacidosis can also occur because of SGLT2 inhibitor use, but typically under specific circumstances or if used off label in patients with type 1 diabetes mellitus.[9]

There are several drug and test interactions that may occur with SGLT2 inhibitors. Urinary glucose is likely to be detected in patients on these drug therapies due to their mechanism of action but should not be a cause for concern. Patients who are on diuretics and SGLT2 inhibitors may have an increased risk of hypotension and acute kidney injury due to dehydration. If there is concern about overdiuresis, one may consider decreasing the dose of the diuretic during initiation of the SGLT2 inhibitor.[9] Canagliflozin has a few additional drug interactions including phenobarbital, phenytoin, rifampin, and ritonavir.[10]

Special Considerations

Weight loss

Some diabetes medications are preferred in patients who desire or have indications to lose weight. In general, GLP-1 RAs and SGLT2 inhibitors are the preferred agents in this patient population. Metformin and DPP-4 inhibitors are considered weight neutral, whereas sulfonylureas and thiazolidinediones should be avoided in patients who need to lose weight because they frequently cause weight gain.[11]

The American Diabetes Association (ADA) Standards of Care suggests initiating a GLP-1 RA early in the T2DM treatment course of patients who could benefit from weight loss.[11] Use of any GLP-1 RA has the potential to result in weight loss in a patient with T2DM. There are also some GLP-1 RA therapies that have been developed and marketed specifically for weight loss in the presence or absence of diabetes: Saxenda (liraglutide) and Wegovy (semaglutide). Without a diagnosis of T2DM, liraglutide and semaglutide can be used in patients who have a body mass index (BMI) greater than or equal to 30 kg/m^2 or in those with BMI of greater than or equal to 27 kg/m^2 and a weight-related comorbidity. The amount of weight loss varies between treatments with studies of liraglutide showing a 6% weight loss and semaglutide having more than 9% weight loss when used in combination with lifestyle interventions. Several studies have investigated whether the weight loss seen with GLP-1 RAs is sustainable, and most have found that the weight lost during therapy is often gained back when therapy is discontinued.[12]

SGLT2 inhibitors produce moderate weight loss, primarily due to loss of glucose in the urine. SGLT2 inhibitor monotherapy does not provide sufficient weight loss for successful treatment of obesity alone.[13] SGLT2 inhibitors are still recommended by ADA as one of the therapies that should be considered in patients with T2DM who need to avoid gaining weight or could benefit from weight loss.[11]

Cardiovascular disease

Several innovative therapies have recently been shown in clinical trials to have cardiovascular benefits independent of their effects on diabetes. The disease states in which

Table 1
Noninsulin therapies for type 2 diabetes mellitus[2,4,5,7,9–11]

Drug Class	Medications in the Class	When to Use	A_{1c} Reduction	Side Effects and Contraindications	Special Considerations	Cost
Biguanide	Metformin	First line in most patients	1%–1.5%	*Side effects:* diarrhea *Rare, serious:* lactic acidosis *Contraindications:* eGFR <30 mL/min/1.73m^2	Dose adjust for renal dysfunction; can use in pre-DM; use extended release with GI upset	$
Sulfonylureas	Glimepiride, glipizide, glyburide	When cost is a consideration	1%–2%	*Side effects:* hypoglycemia, weight gain	Low cost; dose with mealtimes	$
GLP-1 RA	Dulaglutide (Trulicity), exenatide (Byetta), exenatide ER (Bydureon), liraglutide (Victoza, Saxenda), lixisenatide (Adlyxin), semaglutide (Ozempic, Rybelsus, Wegovy)	When weight loss is desired; when patient has a history of ASCVD	0.8%–1.6%	*Side effects:* GI, pancreatitis *Contraindications:* personal or family history of medullary or C-cell thyroid cancer; MEN2	Decreases appetite; potential for weight loss; low risk of hypoglycemia	$$$
DPP-4 inhibitors	Sitagliptin (Januvia), saxagliptin (Onglyza), linagliptin (Tradjenta), alogliptin (Nesina, Vipidia)	When patient is poorly compliant with multiple daily dosing options, resistant to injections	0.6%–0.8%	*Side effects:* Nasopharyngitis, skin lesions, joint pain	Weight neutral; low risk of hypoglycemia; saxagliptin may increase risk of hospitalization due to HF; dose adjustment needed for some in renal dysfunction; do not use in combination with GLP-1 RA; good tolerability and safety profile	$$$

(*continued on next page*)

Table 1
(continued)

Drug Class	Medications in the Class	When to Use	A_{1c} Reduction	Side Effects and Contraindications	Special Considerations	Cost
SGLT-2 inhibitors	Empagliflozin (Jardiance), dapagliflozin (Farxiga), canagliflozin (Invokana)	When patient has a history of HF or CKD; when weight loss is desired	0.5%–0.7%	*Side effects:* GU fungal infection, UTI, Fournier gangrene, hypotension, fracture risk	Benefits in HF and CKD	$$$
Thiazolidinediones	Pioglitazone	When cost is a consideration	0.5%–1.4%	*Side effects:* fluid retention; weight gain; fractures *Contraindications:* pregnancy, bladder cancer, heart failure	High side effect profile; should thoroughly weigh risks vs benefits prior to use	$$

Abbreviations: $, Around $4 for 1 month supply; $$, $10–$20 for a 1-month supply; $$$, more than $100 for a 1-month supply; ASCVD, atherosclerotic cardiovascular disease; CKD, chronic kidney disease; DM, diabetes mellitus; eGFR, estimated glomerular filtration rate; HF, heart failure; GI, gastrointestinal; genitourinary; GU; UTI, urinary tract infections.

they show benefit and their benefit in relation to presence or absence of diabetes depends on the medication class and the drug within the class.

GLP-1 RAs as a class have been shown to have positive effects on cardiovascular outcomes. Subcutaneous semaglutide has improved outcomes, primarily in nonfatal stroke and cardiac revascularization in patients who are at high cardiovascular risk.[14] Liraglutide showed lower rates of death from cardiovascular causes and myocardial infarction.[15] Dulaglutide showed a decreased incidence of stroke, but no significant changes in other cardiovascular outcomes.[16] Lixisenatide, weekly exenatide, and oral semaglutide have shown no benefits in patients with underlying cardiovascular disease, but do not worsen outcomes in these patients.[17]

SGLT2 inhibitors have also shown cardiovascular benefit as a class. Empagliflozin showed a decrease in death from cardiovascular causes and hospitalization for heart failure.[18,19] Dapagliflozin and canagliflozin both showed a decrease in hospitalization for heart failure but did not show significant reductions in any other areas.[20,21] As a result of these studies, empagliflozin and dapagliflozin are now indicated for treatment of patients with heart failure, independent of their diabetes status.

Chronic kidney disease

Many patients with diabetes develop concomitant chronic kidney disease (CKD). Renal protective effects have been seen with SGLT2 inhibitors, and some have gained indications for preserving kidney function. Dapagliflozin has shown consistent benefits in preserving kidney function in patients with and without diabetes.[22] Canagliflozin also slows the progression of kidney disease in patients with T2DM.[23] It is important to note that although SGLT2 inhibitors are beneficial in preserving kidney function, they have a less pronounced effect on glucose control as kidney function worsens. An initial decrease in glomerular filtration rate (GFR) is anticipated with initiation of SGLT2 inhibitors, with benefits seen in long-term preservation of kidney function.[23]

Adherence considerations

Most patients with T2DM require multiple therapies to maintain glucose levels and HbA_{1c} within target ranges. High pill burdens can be a barrier to compliance in many patients. Several diabetes therapies are available in combination to alleviate some of these concerns. SGLT2 inhibitors and DPP-4 inhibitors are available in combination with metformin. One can also find SGLT2 inhibitors with DPP-4 inhibitors in 1 tablet.

Route of administration may also be a barrier to adherence in some patients. GLP-1 RAs are very effective therapies for treatment of T2DM, but patients who are averse to using needles may be hesitant to use these therapies. In late 2019, semaglutide became the first and only oral GLP-1 RA on the market that has the potential to alleviate concerns of injections while preserving the benefits of the drug class.

Cost considerations

With newer drug therapies on the market, considering the cost and insurance coverage of therapies is important during patient care. All SGLT2 inhibitors, DPP-4 inhibitors, and GLP-1 RAs are currently only available in brand name formulations. Within insurance company formularies, most will have a preferred drug within the class. For those who are uninsured, these therapies are not accessible for most unless they are able to use assistance programs through drug manufacturers.

The most cost-effective therapies available for T2DM are metformin, sulfonylureas, and thiazolinediones.[11] In patients who do not have insurance or are unable to afford brand name therapies, these may be considered in their care. Metformin is used first line in most patients, but there are disadvantages to consider in the other cost-effective treatments available. Sulfonylureas can cause significant weight gain and hypoglycemia, whereas thiazolinediones should be used with caution in patients who are at risk for developing congestive heart failure.

Insulin for Type 2 Diabetes Mellitus

Although treatment of T2DM typically starts with noninsulin therapies, most patients progress to insulin dependence through the course of their disease. Generally, insulin will be initiated with basal therapies first, followed by bolus therapies as needed for postprandial coverage.[11] Currently available insulin therapies can be found in **Table 2**.

Basal, or long-acting, insulins are started once daily in most cases; they can be dosed morning or evening but need to be given at the same time each day. Long-acting insulin's onset of action occurs in approximately 2 hours and lasts up to 24 hours. Advantages of long-acting insulins are their long timing of action as well as their lack of a peak, giving a steady rate of blood glucose lowering over time. Insulin degludec is the only ultra-long-acting insulin with an onset of 6 hours and duration of action of at least 36 hours.[24]

Rapid-acting, or bolus, insulins are typically dosed at mealtime in patients with T2DM. Rapid-acting insulins have onset of action in 15 minutes, and therefore should be administered 5 to 15 minutes before a meal. The peak occurs about 1 hour after administration, and they last between 2 and 4 hours.[24] Regular, or short-acting insulin is most like rapid acting insulin, but onset of action is slower and timex to peak is longer. This insulin can be used as a mealtime insulin but should be taken 15 to 30 minutes before eating. Intermediate-acting insulin (NPH insulin) has an onset of action of 2 to 4 hours and has a varied peak, between 4 and 12 hours. This product is often dosed twice daily due to its 12- to-18-h duration of action.[24] In addition to insulin with individual components, mixed insulins are also available. These products contain a longer-acting insulin analogue and a rapid-acting insulin. Alternately, mixed insulins are also available in a combination of NPH insulin and regular insulin.

There have been advancements in insulin therapies over the last several years, including the introduction of concentrated and biosimilar insulins. Historically, all insulins came as 100 units/mL. In the last several years, manufacturers have developed various products that come in a concentrated formulation. In these cases, the insulins come in concentrations of 200 to 500 units/mL. In a scenario when a patient is using this type of insulin, they are required to inject lower volumes of insulin to receive the same dose. Some of the concentrated insulins on the market include insulin glargine U-300 (Toujeo), insulin lispro U-200 lispro (Humalog), and insulin degludec U-200 (Tresiba). The primary reason to choose a concentrated insulin over a nonconcentrated formulation is when patients are taking large volumes of insulin that may be more painful.[25]

A biosimilar product is defined as a biological medicine that has no clinical difference in safety, quality, or efficacy in treatment. Biosimilar products can be considered for manufacturing when a patent has run out on a branded drug product. Although costs are reduced, they are not reduced as much as one may see in a generic medication due to the increased complexity of the manufacturing and approval process.[23] Follow-on products are also newly available. These products differ from biosimilars due to their approval process but may be considered biosimilars in some other countries. The United States currently has 1 biosimilar product on the market (insulin glargine-yfgn, Semglee) and 2 follow-on insulin products (insulin glargine, Basaglar; insulin lispro, Admelog).[26,27]

Cost of insulin can be a significant barrier for many patients. The introduction of biosimilars has aided and will continue to aid in making insulin more attainable for patients

Table 2
Insulin products[24]

Insulin	Products Available	Timing of Action	Concentration (units/mL)
Insulin aspart	Novolog Fiasp	Rapid	U-100
Insulin glargine	Apidra	Rapid	U-100
Insulin lispro	Admelog Humalog Lyumjev	Rapid	U-100, U-200
Human regular insulin	Humulin R Novolin R ReliOn R	Regular	U-100 U-500
NPH insulin	Humulin N Novolin N ReliOn N	Intermediate	U-100
Insulin degludec	Tresiba	Ultra-long	U-100, U-200
Insulin detemir	Levemir	Long	U-100
Insulin glargine	Basaglar Lantus Toujeo	Long	U-100 U-100 U-300
Mixed insulin	Humulin/Novolin 70/30 Humulin/Novolin 50/50 Novolog 70/30 Humalog 70/30 Humalog 50/50	Mixed	U-100

with limited income or lack of insurance coverage. In addition, NPH and regular insulin are available as over-the-counter products, with some being available for a discounted price. These discounted insulins are only available at certain pharmacies and may assist patients who are having affordability problems.

Course of Treatment

When initiating treatment of T2DM, clinicians should start metformin or consider the patient's comorbidities, which may help direct treatment and improve outcomes in all disease states considered. For patients who are on limited income and with little or no insurance coverage, sulfonylureas or thiazolinediones should be considered as second-line therapy, after metformin.[11]

GLP-1 RAs have a prominent role in therapy for treatment of T2DM, being used second line in many patients and the potential to be used first line in patients with certain compelling indications. GLP-1 RAs are appropriate options in patients at high risk for or with known atherosclerotic cardiovascular disease (ASCVD). In patients with T2DM who are desiring weight loss, GLP-1 RAs are the drug of choice; they are also good add-on options for patients with CKD who are already on an SGLT2 inhibitor but have not achieved their glycemic goal. In most cases, GLP-1 RAs should be considered before the initiation of insulin therapy. In patients with T2DM in whom insulin has already been initiated, addition of a GLP-1 RA is still beneficial in most patients.[11]

SGLT2 inhibitors are indicated in patients with T2DM who also have heart failure, ASCVD, or CKD regardless of baseline HbA_{1c} due to proven benefits in patients with these comorbidities. SGLT-2 inhibitor use in these patient populations can be done as initial therapy or as add-on therapy to metformin, depending on the clinician's preference.[11] Insulin therapy is used in T2DM treatment when noninsulin therapies are not sufficient to meet glycemic goals. There are some instances when one would consider initiating insulin early in therapy for a patient with T2DM, and this includes when there is ongoing weight loss, continued symptoms of hyperglycemia, or when HbA_{1c} is more than 10% or blood glucose readings are more than 300 mg/dL.[11]

DPP-4 inhibitors have a less prominent role in therapy than the previous therapies discussed, but should still be used in certain scenarios, such as patients who are at risk for hypoglycemia and patients who need to avoid weight gain. Traditionally, DPP-4 inhibitors should be avoided in combination with GLP-1 RAs due to their similar mechanism of action and lack of significant HbA_{1c} reduction when combined.[11]

Clinical Scenarios

An obese 64-year-old woman presents with HbA_{1c} of 8.7% and a desire to lose weight. She is currently compliant with metformin 1000 mg orally twice a day. She has no other known comorbidities.

What could you add next?

GLP-1 RA

She has a fear of needles and refuses any injectables. What now?

That's ok! Semaglutide has an oral option (Rybelsus)

A 61-year-old obese man with a history of heart failure with reduced ejection fraction (HFrEF) presents with HbA_{1c} of 8.2%. He is currently compliant with metformin 1000 mg orally twice a day.

What could you add next?

SGLT2 inhibitor

A 58-year-old woman with stage 3A CKD (estimated GFR of 49 mL/min/1.73 m^2) presents with HbA_{1c} of 8.4%. She is currently compliant with metformin 1000 mg orally twice a day.

What should you add next?

SGLT2 inhibitor

A 52-year-old man with BMI of 24 kg/m^2 presents with HbA_{1c} of 7.9%. He is compliant with his metformin XR 1000 mg once daily and lifestyle modifications. He has difficulty with compliance if his medications are dosed more frequently, and he prefers to avoid injectables. He also prefers to take as few tablets per day as possible. He has no comorbidities.

What changes could be made in this scenario to help your patient reach his goal HbA_{1c} while still encouraging compliance?

Discontinue his current metformin XR and start *Janumet XR.*

A 67-year-old obese woman with a known history of ASCVD is diagnosed in your clinic today with new-onset T2DM. She has been unsuccessful with her attempts to diet and exercise since her previous provider told her that she had prediabetes 1 year ago. Her HbA_{1c} today is 9.2%.

What should you start this patient on today?

GLP-1 RA

SUMMARY

In summary, it is easy to see why clinicians may be initially overwhelmed when it comes to implementing diabetes management guidelines, especially when managing complex patients with multiple comorbidities. This article provides a summary of compelling indications and special considerations for some of the more recent innovations in diabetes management in hopes of making clinical application of diabetes management guidelines less intimidating. This in turn, will encourage more aggressive management of T2DM so that progress will be made in attaining the goals set by Healthy People 2023.

CLINICS CARE POINTS

- GLP-1 RAs have proven benefits in patients with T2DM with a history of cardiovascular disease and typically also result in weight loss.
  - Good initial therapy, second-line therapy, or used in combination with insulin
  - Most are injectables
  - Avoid in patients with personal or family history of medullary or C-cell thyroid cancer or MEN2
- DPP-4 inhibitors have proven benefits in glycemic control.
  - No effect on weight
  - Well tolerated
  - Avoid in combination with GLP-1 RAs due to similar mechanism of action
- SGLT-2 inhibitors have proven benefits in patients with heart failure and CKD and have the added benefit of weight loss.
  - Urinary excretion of glucose leads to increased genitourinary infection risk
  - Empagliflozin and dapagliflozin indicated in patients with heart failure, regardless of diabetes status
  - Although proved to have long-term benefits in CKD, they may initially cause transient decrease in GFR
- Thiazolinediones have a high side effect profile, and their use should be reserved for certain situations when the benefits have been determined to outweigh the risks.
  - Fluid retention, heart failure
  - Weight gain
  - Affordable option
- Sulfonylureas also have more limited use in the management of diabetes due to the many therapeutic options available today.
  - Weight gain
  - Affordable option

DISCLOSURE

Neither author has any commercial or financial conflicts of interest to disclose.

REFERENCES

1. U.S. Department of Health and Human Services. Healthy People 2030. Available at: https://health.gov/healthypeople. Accessed June 22, 2022.
2. Hinnen D. Glucagon-like peptide 1 receptor agonists for type 2 diabetes. Diabetes Spectr 2017;30(3):202–10.
3. Drucker DJ. Mechanisms of action and therapeutic application of glucagon-like peptide-1. Cell Metab 2018;27(4):740–56.
4. Semaglutide. Lexi-Drugs. Hudson (OH): Lexicomp; 2022. Available at: http://online.lexi.com/. Accessed April 2022.
5. Liraglutide. Lexi-Drugs. Hudson (OH): Lexicomp; 2022. Available at: http://online.lexi.com/. Accessed April 2022.
6. Gomez-Peralta F, Abreu C, Gomez-Rodriguez S, et al. Safety and efficacy of DPP4 inhibitor and basal insulin in type 2 diabetes: an updated review and challenging clinical scenarios. Diabetes Ther 2018;9(5):1775–89.

7. Sitagliptin. Lexi-Drugs. Hudson (OH): Lexicomp; 2022. Available at: http://online.lexi.com. Accessed April 2022.
8. Mikhail N. Place of sodium-glucose co-transporter type 2 inhibitors for treatment of type 2 diabetes. World J Diabetes 2014;5(6):854–9.
9. Empagliflozin. Lexi-Drugs. Hudson (OH): Lexicomp; 2022. Available at: http://online.lexi.com/. Accessed April 2022.
10. Canagliflozin. Lexi-Drugs. Hudson (OH): Lexicomp; 2022. Available at: http://online.lexi.com/. Accessed April 2022.
11. American Diabetes Association. Standards of medical care in diabetes – 2022. Diabetes Care 2021;45. https://doi.org/10.2337/dc22-Sint.
12. Rubino D, Abrahamsson N, Davies M, et al. Effect of continued weekly subcutaneous semaglutide vs placebo on weight loss maintenance in adults with overweight or obesity: the STEP 4 randomized clinical trial. J Am Med Assoc 2021;325(14):1414–25.
13. Zheng Hanrui, Liu Min, Li Sheyu, et al. Sodium-glucose co-transporter-2 inhibitors in non-diabetic adults with overweight or obesity: a systematic review and meta-analysis. Front Endocrinol (Lausanne) 2021;12. https://doi.org/10.3389/fendo.2021.706914.
14. Marso SP, Bain SC, Consoli A, et al. Semaglutide and cardiovascular outcomes in patients with type 2 diabetes. N Engl J Med 2016;375:1834–44.
15. Marso SP, Daniels GH, Brown-Frandsen K, et al. Liraglutide and cardiovascular outcomes in type 2 diabetes. N Engl J Med 2016;375:311–22.
16. Gerstein HC, Colhoun HM, Dagenais GR, et al. Dulaglutide and cardiovascular outcomes in type 2 diabetes (REWIND): a double-blind, randomized placebo-controlled trial. Lancet 2019;394(10193):121–30.
17. Sheahan KH, Wahlberg EA, Gilbert MP. An overview of GLP-1 agonists and recent cardiovascular outcomes trials. Postgrad Med J 2020;96:156–61.
18. Zinman B, Wanner C, Lachin JM, et al. Empagliflozin, cardiovascular outcomes, and mortality in type 2 diabetes. N Engl J Med 2015;373:2117–28.
19. Anker SD, Butler J, Filippatos G, et al. Empagliflozin in heart failure with a preserved ejection fraction. N Engl J Med 2021;385:1451–61.
20. Wiviott SD, Raz I, Bonaca MP, et al. Dapagliflozin and cardiovascular outcomes in type 2 diabetes. N Engl J Med 2019;380:347–57.
21. Neal B, Perkovic V, Mahaffey KW, et al. Canagliflozin and cardiovascular and renal events in type 2 diabetes. N Engl J Med 2017;377:644–57.
22. Heerspink HJL, Stefansson BV, Correa-Rotter R, et al. Dapagliflozin in patients with chronic kidney disease. N Engl J Med 2020;383:1436–46.
23. Perkovic V, Jardine MJ, Neal B, et al. Canagliflozin and renal outcomes in type 2 diabetes and nephropathy. N Engl J Med 2019;380:2295–306.
24. Center for Disease Control and Prevention. Types of insulin. Available at: https://www.cdc.gov/diabetes/basics/type-1-types-of-insulin.html. Accessed June 22, 2022.
25. Gonzalvo JD, Patel DK, Olin JL. Concentrated insulins: a review and recommendations. Fed Pract 2017;34(Suppl 8):S38–43.
26. Morris D. Biosimilar insulins: an in-depth guide. J Diabetes Nurs 2022;26(1):228.
27. White J, Wagner A, Patel H. The impact of biosimilar insulins on the diabetes landscape. J Manag Care Spec Pharm 2022;28(1):91–8.

Therapeutic Benefits of Medical Cannabis

Emily R. Hajjar, PharmD, MS, BCPS, BCACP, BCGP[a,*], Jessica M. Lungen, PharmD Candidate[a], Brooke K. Worster, MD[b]

KEYWORDS

• Cannabis • Tetrahydrocannabinol (THC) • Cannabidiol (CBD) • Cannabinoid

KEY POINTS

- The 2 most-studied cannabinoids are tetrahydrocannabinol (THC) and cannabidiol.
- Therapeutic uses for cannabis can include pain, insomnia, anxiety, and nausea/anorexia.
- Most troubling side effects are related to concentration of THC in various product forms.
- There are many pharmacokinetic and pharmacodynamic drug–drug interactions associated with the use of cannabis.

INTRODUCTION

Despite the increase in the use of medical cannabis, the science of cannabis falls seriously behind state cannabis laws and clinical practice and national guidelines lack recommendations on cannabis use.[1–3] Although cannabis is still federally classified as a Schedule I substance by the US Food and Drug Administration, at least 36 states and the District of Columbia have approved cannabis for medical use and 18 others have laws allowing legal recreational access.[4] Recent epidemiologic surveys evaluating trajectories of cannabis use as a function of the changing policy landscape have revealed rates of cannabis use by adults aged 18 years and older in the United States have increased overall.[5]

The term "medical" cannabis involves using the natural, dried plant material, which includes the flower buds, stems, and leaves or extracts of the cannabis plant for health, wellness, or symptom palliation. Additionally, this term does involve the use of synthetic or prescription whole plant extracts that can have effects similar to that of medical cannabis. Generally, medical cannabis is obtained from a dispensary through a certification process. Although laws vary from state to state, patients are

[a] Jefferson College of Pharmacy, Thomas Jefferson University, 901 Walnut Street, Suite 901, Philadelphia, PA 19107, USA; [b] Division of Supportive Oncology, Sidney Kimmel Medical College, Thomas Jefferson University, 925 Chestnut Street, 5th Floor, Philadelphia, PA 19107, USA
* Corresponding author. 901 Walnut Street, Suite 901, Philadelphia, PA 19107.
E-mail address: Emily.hajjar@jefferson.edu

Physician Assist Clin 8 (2023) 281–291
https://doi.org/10.1016/j.cpha.2022.10.008

certified based on a medical condition, which allows them to access various cannabis products. This differs from a prescriptive process because patients may rely on a medical professional or cannabis staff member at the dispensary for product selection as opposed to the practitioner who certifies them. Patients may also choose to use cannabis that they purchase outside of dispensary locations for both medicinal and recreational purposes, and although they may experience similar effects to medical cannabis, there is no reliable way to know what is contained in the substances purchased in nondispensary locations. There are some data that show serious side effects related to "medically" regulated cannabis use are less than illicit cannabis, likely due to the unknown composition of cannabis purchased outside of regulated sources.[6]

Understanding the terminology associated with cannabis is an important foundation for educational awareness related to its composition, safety, or availability. The US government created the distinction between "high" (>0.3% tetrahydrocannabinol [THC]) and "low" THC (<0.3% THC) cannabis as a regulatory mechanism. This does not serve as a medical or scientific distinction but rather a mechanism of legislation. The Farm Bill of 2018 deregulated "low" THC cannabis, known as hemp (**Table 1**).[7] Inappropriately, due to the low amounts of THC, hemp may be referred to as cannabidiol (CBD), although this nomenclature is inaccurate, because hemp can contain numerous phytochemical compounds, including THC. Subsequently due to the deregulation of hemp, innumerable CBD-based products flooded the marketplace with little to no regulation in content or quality.[8] Although patients have online or even convenience store access to these CBD products, there is minimal assurance of quality or composition.

Pharmacology and Adverse Effects

Although there are many cannabinoids (CBs) found in cannabis, CBD and THC are the most widely studied components. Cannabis exhibits effects through the CB receptors CB1 and CB2. CB1 receptors are primarily found on the neurons in the central nervous system as well as on some peripheral targets such as within the cardiovascular system and within the gastrointestinal tract. The CB2 receptors are primarily located in the periphery, and expressed when there is an active inflammation, on immune cells as well as within the spleen and tonsillar tissue.[9,10] THC is a partial agonist of both receptors but it is through the CB1 receptor that its psychoactive effects are seen. CBD has a

Table 1
Components of marijuana and hemp products

United States Law Defines as:	Marijuana[a]	Hemp	Synthetic (Dronabinol)
Plant components	Leaves, flowers, and viable seeds of cannabis	Stalks, stems, and sterilized seeds of cannabis	None
Δ9-THC = main psychoactive component	>0.3%	<0.3%	Individual capsules or liquid with 5 mg synthetic THC
CBD	Any	Any	None

Cannabis, taxonomic term referring to a genus of flowering plants that are members of the family Cannabaceae, consisting of 1000s of phytochemicals, divided into 3 species (*Cannabis sativa*, *Cannabis indica*, *Cannabis ruderalis*).

[a] Used interchangeably with cannabis, given range of possible patient products used, term cannabis is more accurate and inclusive in this setting.

low affinity for the CB1 and CB2 receptors and acts as a noncompetitive negative allosteric modulator of the CB1 receptor. CBD can inhibit THC binding at the CB1 receptor and can also bind to other non-CB receptors.[11] Stimulation of the CB1 receptor results in reduction in motor activity, sedation, and pain relief, whereas stimulation of the CB2 receptor leads to pain relief and anti-inflammatory actions.[12]

Cannabis consumption through any formulation can lead to side effects such as dry mouth, dizziness, sedation, euphoria, headache, appetite stimulation, and cognitive impairment. These side effects are primarily related to the THC component and are known to be dose dependent and may be minimized if doses are slowly titrated to effect.[13] Less common side effects include psychosis, depression, ataxia, tachycardia, orthostasis, diarrhea, and cannabis hyperemesis syndrome (CHS).[13] Although many adverse effects are unwanted, some side effects associated with cannabis can be used in a beneficial way such as those with insomnia may benefit from its side effect of sedation or a person with anorexia may benefit from its side effect of appetite stimulation.

If cannabis is used at high doses for prolonged periods, CHS can develop. CHS symptoms include cycles of nausea, vomiting, and abdominal pain, which can be immediately relieved by bathing in hot water.[14] When cannabis is consumed during a long period of time, abrupt discontinuation can lead to side effects of cannabis withdrawal. Common symptoms that occur during cannabis withdrawal are anxiety, depression, sleep difficulty, aggression, or decreased appetite.[15]

Cannabis Dosage Forms and Pharmacokinetics

Cannabis is available in inhalation, oral, sublingual, and topical formulations that vary in terms of their pharmacokinetic properties. Choice of dosage form is based on patient preference and the desired therapeutic onset and duration of action (**Table 2**).

Inhalation

Inhalation is the most common way in which cannabis is ingested and the effects of cannabis can be experienced quickly so patients may find inhalational products easiest to titrate to effect. To inhale cannabis, the raw flower or concentrates can be used. Although smoking cannabis is popular, it is not recommended, and in some states, it is required that medical cannabis be vaporized, not smoked. When smoking cannabis, the product needs to be combusted to a temperature between 600°C and 900°C.[13] However, when the product is vaporized, it is only heated to 160°C to 230°C and the vapor is inhaled.[13] The lower temperature decreases the production of toxic byproducts as well as pulmonary symptoms. Although smoked or vaporized medical cannabis is popular, it has a relatively short duration of action and may need to be consumed multiple times per day if a sustained effect is needed.[13]

Table 2
Cannabis pharmacokinetics[10,11,44–46]

Dosage Form	Onset	Peak	Duration
Inhalation	0–10 min	3–10 min	2–4 h
Oral	30 min–2 h	1–2 h	6–12 h
Sublingual	15–60 min	45 min	4–6 h
Topical	5–120 min	Variable	Variable

Oral/Sublingual

Cannabis can also be ingested through the oral route through oils, capsules, or edible products such as cannabis infused candy, food products, or beverages. Oral administration is becoming more popular due to the longer duration of action but the delayed onset of effect can make dosing challenging.[13] Patients may be unaware of this delay in onset and take more than the intended dose assuming that the product is not working, which can lead to symptoms of over ingestion and overdose.[16] The recommended approach when initiating cannabis is to start low, go slow. Another consideration of edible cannabis is to keep all products secured because many are formulated in cookies or candies, increasing risk that children and pets can accidently ingest it.[17] Nonfood-based formulations, such as sublingual tinctures can be used and are considered when a longer duration of action is warranted. Sublingual products are placed under the tongue and have a faster onset compared with other oral products.

Topical

Topical products such as oils, patches, creams, and lotions are also available for patients who would prefer to use cannabis for localized disease states such as arthritis or a dermatologic condition.[13] Topical administration limits the systemic effects of cannabis and allows the drug to be delivered over a prolonged period to a localized area. Use of topical cannabis may be associated with local skin irritation but may be preferred for those wanting pain relief without any of the psychoactive adverse effects.[18]

Rick Simpson Oil

Rick Simpson Oil (RSO) products are full-spectrum extracts that are generally high in THC content. These potent products have a viscous consistency and are often supplied in oral syringes. RSO products can be ingested orally, sublingually, or applied topically.[19] Although RSO products have the same considerations as inhalational, oral, and sublingual products, users should note the high potency of the products in order to prevent an unintentional overdose. RSO may also be applied topically for skin cancer treatment, although this is only supported by anecdotal evidence.[19]

Drug–Drug Considerations

Although some may view the use of medical cannabis as a natural product with little risk, it is associated with both pharmacokinetic and pharmacodynamic drug–drug interactions. Pharmacokinetic drug interactions are primarily mediated by the cytochrome P450 enzyme systems, and pharmacodynamic drug interactions are seen when cannabis is used with other medications that produce the same physiologic effect resulting in an additive or synergistic effect. It is important to note that cannabis can affect other medications and other medications can affect the levels of both THC and CBD. Please refer to **Tables 3–5** for more detailed information. Given the many medications that could potentially interact with medical cannabis, it is important to obtain a baseline medication history before initiating cannabis.

Select Clinical Indications

Many clinical uses for cannabis exist as evidenced by the various indications approved by each state for medical use but common reasons for use include pain, insomnia, anxiety, nausea, and anorexia.

Table 3
Cytochrome P450 interactions: effects on medical cannabis[44,47,48]

Enzyme	Medication Examples	Effect
CYP 2C9 inhibitor	Amiodarone, metronidazole, fluoxetine, fluconazole, voriconazole	Potential ↑ effect of cannabis
CYP 2C9 inducer	Barbiturates, carbamazepine, phenytoin	Potential ↓ in the effect of cannabis
CYP 3A4 inhibitor	Ketoconazole, itraconazole, clarithromycin, diltiazem, ritonavir, verapamil	Potential ↑ effect of cannabis
CYP 3A4 inducer	Phenobarbital, phenytoin, rifampicin, St. John's Wort	Potential ↓ in the effect of cannabis
CYP2C19 inhibitor	Cimetidine, clopidogrel, efavirenz, omeprazole, fluconazole, fluoxetine	Potential ↑ effect of cannabis
CYP2C19 inducer	Barbiturates, carbamazepine, phenytoin, rifampin, rifapentine, St. John's Wort	Potential ↓ effect of cannabis

Pain

Very few well-done, randomized controlled trials exist examining medical cannabis in patients with cancer pain. However, there has been increasing interest in cannabis use for both cancer and chronic noncancer pain (CNCP) given the lack of safety or tolerability of opioids and other analgesics (kidney disease and nonsteroidal anti-inflammatory drugs, polypharmacy, risk of addiction with controlled substances). Although evidence is mixed, there seems to be a weak indication for cannabis use if standard of care has failed across pain types.[20] Evidence is somewhat better for cancer pain and CNPC than neuropathic pain or postoperative pain.[21] It remains hard to control for route of administration as well as composition of products.

Insomnia

Impaired sleep onset and latency are frequent concerns among patients with cancer and may affect up to 19% of the general population.[22] One very common patient-reported use of cannabis is to treat insomnia. However, research into cannabis use and sleep is very conflicting. There is some evidence that short-term, high-dose CBD may be helpful in decreasing sleep onset and lengthening time asleep possibly

Table 4
Effect of THC and CBD on other medications[7,49]

Medical Cannabis Component	Enzyme	Effect
THC	Inhibitor of CYP 2A6, 2B6, 2C9, 2D6, 3A4	Potential increased effects on affected medication
THC (smoked)	Inducer of CYP 1A1 and 1A2	Potential decrease in levels/ effects on affected medications
CBD	Inhibitor of CYP 2A6, 2B6, 2C8, 2C9, 2C19, 2D6, 3A4	Potential increased effects on affected medication

Table 5
Pharmacodynamic drug interactions with medical cannabis[50]

Medication Class	Medication Example	Effects When Used with THC
Central nervous system (CNS) depressants	Benzodiazepine Alcohol	Sedation Ataxia
Anticholinergic medication	Diphenhydramine	Sedation Tachycardia Confusion
Sympathomimetic agents	Methylphenidate	Tachycardia Hypertension

through its anxiolytic effects.[23,24] Conflicting evidence suggests that cannabis cessation after prolonged use can cause or exacerbate insomnia.[25]

Chronic pain affects individuals' ability to get restful sleep. Research, primarily with nabiximols (Sativex, a 1:1 THC:CBD oromucosal spray), has started to examine the potential role of CBs in addressing sleep disturbances in the context of pain. A significant majority of study patients reported a subjective improvement in sleep quality, although possibly more related to reduced pain levels than a change in biological sleep patterns. Frequent cannabis use, especially high THC products results in tolerance and may trigger self-titration and very high THC use during prolonged exposure for sleep.[26]

Anxiety

Anxiety disorders, as a group, are the most common mental illness in the world, leading to high psychosocial and financial burden.[27] The first-line treatment of anxiety disorders includes various antidepressants (selective serotonin reuptake inhibitors, serotonin norepinephrine reuptake inhibitors) and benzodiazepines as well as psychotherapy. Up to 40% of patients still experience anxiety symptoms despite this treatment, thus driving interest in additional effective therapeutics.[28] CBD has therapeutic potential as a treatment of anxiety as shown by the burgeoning number of studies and meta-analysis examining use in several anxiety disorders, ranging from post-traumatic stress disorder (PTSD) to public speaking. There are well-supported data that high THC can exacerbate anxiety, induce panic attacks or even trigger transient psychosis in nonfrequent users or if overingested, whereas CBD has shown tolerability and effectiveness in social anxiety, PTSD, and general anxiety treatment.[29,30] Studies have looked at both oral and inhaled forms of CBD predominant cannabis with somewhat equal efficacy.

Nausea and Anorexia

There are 2 FDA-approved delta-9-THC pharmaceutical agents, dronabinol and nabilone, for use in treating nausea and vomiting associated with cytotoxic chemotherapy. A meta-analysis summarizing 28 trials, most completed before 2000, favored these over placebo or other antiemetics available.[31] Additional studies completed more recently also support that although patients reported more frequent side effects, they preferred CBs over other antiemetics.[32] Very few trials have examined the influence of CBD alone or CBD predominant cannabis formulations in this setting.

Similarly, patients often subjectively report improvements in appetite with cannabis use. Marinol originally received FDA approval for this indication in HIV patients in the 1980s. Studies show that smoked cannabis increase blood levels of ghrelin and leptin, hormones associated with hunger.[33] Small trials of THC supplementation in patients with advanced cancer have shown subjective reports of improved taste and appetite.[34] Again, there are minimal data focusing on CBD predominant products in appetite stimulation or weight gain.

It is important to note that of all the antiemetics on the market, cannabis or corticosteroids are the only products with both antiemetic and orexigenic effects. However, the risk of elevated blood sugars, infection, or bone health may limit the prolonged use of steroids.

Risks and Contraindications

It is important to consider risks and side effects of cannabis use when counseling patients. Cannabis smoke carries many of the same carcinogens found in tobacco smoke. However, large cross-sectional and longitudinal studies have not found a link between cannabis smoking and long-term pulmonary consequences, such as chronic obstructive pulmonary disease and lung cancer.[35,36] The risks of inhalation as the route of administration often lead many guidelines to steer away from this as a method of consumption.[37]

Recent evidence highlights cardiovascular concerns among cannabis users as well. Randomized controlled trials evaluating the therapeutic use and safety of marijuana are lacking but a growing body of evidence suggests that marijuana consumption may be associated with adverse cardiovascular risks.[38] CB1 receptors are found in the myocardium, aorta, and vasculature; therefore, some interaction between cannabis use and cardiac events is not entirely surprising. There is much to be learned, and most studies now are retrospective analyses with confounding variable such as high prevalence of tobacco use in the populations as well.[39]

One recent study examining the incidence and effect of marijuana use on admissions for patients with prior myocardial infarction (MI) or revascularization procedures from a national inpatient sample during 7 years found an increasing trend of cannabis use with higher rates of acute MI, percutaneous coronary intervention, and coronary artery bypass grafting.[40] Subsequent acute MI was also higher in marijuana users than nonusers (67% vs 41%) in this same population.

Data regarding the relationship between cannabis use and psychiatric disorders are incompletely understood, in conflict, and related to CB type, with synthetic, illicit THC products carrying a much higher risk than whole plant or extract.[41] Although there is a clear association between cannabis use and psychotic disorder, a causal link has yet to be unequivocally established. However, the rate of psychiatric hospitalization is increased in bipolar disorder and schizophrenia patients who use cannabis heavily.[41]

Cannabis Use Disorder

Cannabis use disorder (CUD) is a defined in the Diagnostic and Statistical Manual-fifth edition as, "a problematic pattern of cannabis use leading to clinically significant impairment or distress, occurring within a 12 month period."[15] Common symptoms of CUD include cravings and the persistent desire for and consuming larger amounts of cannabis, impairment in social or occupational functioning due to cannabis and withdrawal.[15] When cannabis is used frequently and for a long duration of time, cessation can lead to symptoms of withdrawal. Approximately 76.3% of people going through cannabis withdrawal experienced nervousness/anxiety, 68.2% had sleep difficulty, 71.9% had hostility, and 58.9% experienced depressed mood.[42] Significant side effects can occur when cannabis is overdosed or overused including lethargy, dizziness, confusion, and drowsiness.[43]

Table 6
Initial THC dosing[13,51]

Form	Dose	Comments
Vaporization/Smoking	1 short inhalation	• Wait 10–15 min to see effect • Inhale longer duration puff for stronger effect
Oral	2.5–5 mg THC/dose	• Consider starting with one-fourth to one-half of edible product • Wait 1–2 h to see effect before redosing for desired effect • May consider increasing the dose every 2–7 d
Sublingual	2.5–5 mg THC/dose	• Wait 45 min to see effect before redosing for desired effect • May consider increasing the dose every 2–7 d
Topical	Liberal amount to affected area(s)	Do not bathe or swim after topical application

Practical Considerations

When considering the use of cannabis in patients, it is important to understand their past and current level of use to guide patient counseling. Those that are naïve to cannabis should start with low doses and titrate to their desired effect (**Table 6**). If a medical professional is available in dispensaries, patients should be encouraged to consult with those experts for final product selection. Patients should also be counseled to keep products in the original dispensary packaging to ensure products can be identified. Products should also be stored in climate-controlled settings and out of direct sunlight to allow for longer product stability.

When patients choose to use medical cannabis, it should be noted within the medication list to ensure that all practitioners consider this when prescribing other medications. Prescribers should also be aware of changes in status of patients such as when patients need inpatient care, where they are likely not able to use their normal cannabis products. Practitioners should be aware of the signs of cannabis withdrawal and be alert for the need for potential additional medications. An example of this is the need for a sleep medication when patients are not allowed to use cannabis for sleep latency issues.

SUMMARY

The use of medical cannabis is increasing and expected to increase further as more states move to comprehensive medical and recreational access. Although high-level evidence may be lacking, patients may receive beneficial effects on disease states such as pain, anxiety, insomnia, nausea, and anorexia. Practitioners should be aware of the risks and benefits of cannabis and treat its use similar to all other pharmacologic treatments.

DISCLOSURE

Dr E.R. Hajjar receives grant funding from Ethos Cannabis. Dr B.K. Worster receives grant funding from Ethos Cannabis and serves on the Scientific Advisory Board for Pax.

REFERENCES

1. Nugent SM, Meghani SH, Rogal SS, et al. Medical cannabis use among individuals with cancer: An unresolved and timely issue. Cancer 2020;126(9):1832–6.
2. Jeffers AM, Glantz S, Byers A, et al. Sociodemographic characteristics associated with and prevalence and frequency of cannabis use among adults in the US. JAMA Netw Open 2021;4(11):e2136571.
3. NCCN. The NCCN guidelines: adult cancer pain (v.1.). National Comprehensive Cancer Network; 2021. Available at: https://www.nccn.org/professionals/physician_gls/pdf/pain.pdf. Accessed February 19, 2022.
4. National Conference of State Legislatures. Cannabis overview 2021. Available at: https://www.ncsl.org/research/civil-and-criminal-justice/marijuana-overview.aspx. Accessed March 1, 2022.
5. Wall M, Cheslack-Postava K, Hu MC, et al. Nonmedical prescription opioids and pathways of drug involvement in the US: Generational differences. Drug Alcohol Depend 2018;182:103–11.
6. Schlag A K. An evaluation of regulatory regimes of medical cannabis: what lessons can be learned for the UK? Med Cannabis Cannabinoids 2020;3:76–83.
7. Bill Farm. US Department of Agriculture. Available at: https://www.usda.gov/farmbill. Accessed April 22, 2022.
8. Bonn-Miller MO, Loflin MJE, Thomas BF, et al. Labeling Accuracy of Cannabidiol Extracts Sold Online. JAMA 2017;318(17):1708–9.
9. Bie B, Wu J, Foss JF, et al. An overview of the cannabinoid type 2 receptor system and its therapeutic potential. Curr Opin Anaesthesiol 2018;31(4):407–14.
10. Grotenhermen F. Pharmacokinetics and pharmacodynamics of cannabinoids. Clin Pharmacokinet 2003;42:327–60.
11. Lucas CL, Galettis P, Schneider J. The pharmacokinetics and pharmacodynamics of cannabinoids. Br J Clin Pharmacol 2018;84:2477–82.
12. Russo EB, Marcu J. Cannabis Pharmacology: The Usual Suspects and a Few Promising Leads. Adv Pharmacol 2017;80:67–134. Epub 2017 Jun 5. PMID: 28826544.
13. MacCallum CA, Russo EB. Practical considerations in medical cannabis administration and dosing. Eur J Intern Med 2018;49:12–9. Epub 2018 Jan 4. PMID: 29307505.
14. Lewis B, Leach E, Fomum Mugri LB, et al. Community-based study of cannabis hyperemesis syndrome. Am J Emerg Med 2021;45:504–5. Epub 2021 May 24. PMID: 34103168.
15. Diagnostic and statistical manual of mental disorders: DSM-5. 5th ed. American Psychiatric Association; 2013.
16. Grewal JKm Loh LC. Health consideration of the legalization of cannabis edibles. CMAJ 2020;192:E1–2.
17. Barrus DG, Capogrossi KL, Cates SC, et al. Tasty THC: promises and challenges of cannabis edibles. Methods Rep RTI Press; 2016.
18. Casiraghi A, Musazzi UM, Centin G, et al. Topical administration of cannabidiol: influence of vehicle-related aspects on skin permeation process. Pharmaceuticals (Basel) 2020;13(11):337. PMCID: PMC7690861.
19. Romano LL, Hazekamp A. Cannabis Oil: chemical evaluation of an upcoming cannabis-based medicine. Cannabinoids 2013;1(1):1–11.
20. Caulley L. Medical marijuana for chronic pain. N Engl J Med 2018;379(16): 1575–7.

21. McDonagh MS, Wagner J, Ahmed AY, et al. Living systematic review on cannabis and other plant-based treatments for chronic pain. Comparative effectiveness review No. 250. Rockville, MD: Agency for Healthcare Research and Quality; October 2021. https://doi.org/10.23970/AHRQEPCCER250 (Prepared by Pacific Northwest Evidence-based Practice Center under Contract No. 75Q80120D00006.) AHRQ Publication No. 21(22)-EHC036.
22. Davidson JR, MacLean AW, Brundage MD, et al. Sleep disturbance in cancer patients. Soc Sci Med 2002;54(9):1309–21.
23. Carlini EA, Cunha JM, Paulo S. Hypnotic and antiepileptic effects of cannabidiol. J Clin Pharmacol 1981;21:417S–27S.
24. Betthauser K, Pilz J, Vollmer LE. Use and effects of cannabinoids in military veterans with posttraumatic stress disorder. Am J Heal Pharm 2015;72(15):1279–84.
25. Bolla KI, Lesage SR, Gamaldo CE, et al. Sleep disturbance in heavy marijuana users. Sleep 2008;31(6):901–8.
26. Sznitman SR, Vulfsons S, Meiri D, et al. Medical cannabis and insomnia in older adults with chronic pain: A cross-sectional study. BMJ Support Palliat Care 2020; 10(4):415–20.
27. Scherma M, Masia P, Deidda M, et al. New perspectives on the use of cannabis in the treatment of psychiatric disorders. Medicines 2018;5(4):107.
28. Stein MB, Craske MG. Treating anxiety in 2017: optimizing care to improve outcomes. JAMA 2017;318(3):235–6.
29. Lamers CTJ, Bechara A, Rizzo M, et al. Cognitive function and mood in MDMA/THC users, THC users and non-drug using controls. J Psychopharmacol 2006; 20(2):302–11.
30. Wright M, Di Ciano P, Brands B. Use of cannabidiol for the treatment of anxiety: a short synthesis of pre-clinical and clinical evidence. Cannabis Cannabinoid Res 2020;5(3):191–6.
31. Whiting PF, Wolff RF, Deshpande S, et al. Cannabinoids for medical use: a systematic review and meta-analysis. JAMA 2015;313(24):2456–73.
32. Phillips RS, Friend AJ, Gibson F, et al. Antiemetic medication for prevention and treatment of chemotherapy-induced nausea and vomiting in childhood. Cochrane Database Syst Rev 2016;2(2):CD007786. PMID: 26836199; PMCID: PMC7073407.
33. Riggs PK, Vaida F, Rossi SS, et al. A pilot study of the effects of cannabis on appetite hormones in HIV-infected adult men. Brain Res 2012;1431:46–52.
34. Abrams DI, Guzman M. Cannabis in cancer care. Clin Pharmacol Ther 2015; 97(6):575–86.
35. Tashkin DP. Effects of marijuana smoking on the lung. Ann Am Thorac Soc 2013; 10:239–47. 23.
36. Zhang LR, Morgenstern H, Greenland S, et al. Cannabis smoking and lung cancer risk: pooled analysis in the International Lung Cancer Consortium. Int J Cancer 2015;136:894–903.
37. Busse JW, Vankrunkelsven P, Zeng L, et al. Medical cannabis or cannabinoids for chronic pain: A clinical practice guideline. BMJ 2021;374. https://doi.org/10.1136/bmj.n2040.
38. Latif Z, Garg N. The Impact of Marijuana on the Cardiovascular System: A Review of the Most Common Cardiovascular Events Associated with Marijuana Use. J Clin Med 2020;9:1925.
39. Patel RS, Katta SR, Patel R, et al. Cannabis use disorder in young adults with acute myocardial infarction: trend inpatient study from 2010 to 2014 in the United States. Cureus 2018;10:e3241.

40. Desai R, Singh S, Gandhi ZJ, et al. Abstract 15863: Prevalence, trends and impact of cannabis use on hospitalizations with prior myocardial infarction and revascularization. Circulation 2020;142:A15863.
41. Moore TH, Zammit S, Lingford-Hughes A, et al. Cannabis use and risk of psychotic or affective mental health outcomes: a systematic review. Lancet 2007; 370:319–28.
42. Livne O, Shmulewitz D, Lev-Ran S, et al. DSM-5 cannabis withdrawl syndrome: demographics and clinical correlated in US adults. Drug Alcohol Depend 2019; 195:170–7.
43. Noble MJ, Hedberg K, Hendrickson RG. Acute cannabis toxicity. Clin Toxicol (Phila) 2019;57(8):735–42.
44. Foster BC, Abramovici H, Harris CS. Cannabis and Cannabinoids: Kinetics and Interactions. Am J Med 2019;132(11):1266–70. Epub 2019 May 30. PMID: 31152723.
45. Huestis MA. Pharmacokinetics and metabolism of the plant cannabinoids, delta9-tetrahydrocannabinol, cannabidiol and cannabinol. Handb Exp Pharmacol 2005; 168:657–90.
46. Hosseini A, McLachlan AJ, Lickliter JD. A phase I trial of the safety, tolerability and pharmacokinetics of cannabidiol administered as single-dose oil solution and single and multiple doses of a sublingual wafer in healthy volunteers. Br J Clin Pharmacol 2021;87(4):2070–7.
47. Alsherbiny MA, Li CG. Medicinal cannabis—potential drug interactions. Medicines 2019;6(1):3.
48. Brown JD, Winterstein AG. Potential adverse drug events and drug-drug interactions with medical and consumer cannabidiol (CBD) use. J Clin Med 2019;8(7): 989. PMID: 31288397; PMCID: PMC6678684.
49. Yamaori S, Maeda C, Yamamoto I, et al. Differential inhibition of human cytochrome P450 2A6 and 2B6 by major phytocannabinoids. Forensic Toxicol 2011;29:117–24.
50. Antoniou T, Bodkin J, Ho JMW. Drug interactions with cannabinoids. CMAJ 2020; 192:E206.
51. Bhaskar A, Bell A, Boivin M, et al. Consensus recommendations on dosing and administration of medical cannabis to treat chronic pain: results of a modified Delphi process. J Cannabis Res 2021;3(1):22. PMID: 34215346; PMCID: PMC8252988.

Pharmacotherapeutic Management of Hypertensive Crisis

Sarah S. Harlan, PharmD, BCCCP[a], Julie E. Farrar, PharmD, BCCCP[b,*]

KEYWORDS

• Hypertension • Antihypertensive agents • Hypertensive emergency
• Hypertensive urgency

KEY POINTS

- Hypertensive crisis (HTN-C) is a severe increase in blood pressure to greater than 180/120 mm Hg.
- HTN-C can be broken into 2 subcategories including hypertensive emergency (HTN-E; presence of end-organ damage) and hypertensive urgency (HTN-U; absence of end-organ damage).
- Parenteral antihypertensive agents should be used in HTN-E to lower blood pressure by 20% to 25% in the first hour unless otherwise guided by end-organ disease.
- Patients presenting with HTN-U should receive oral antihypertensives to decrease blood pressure to outpatient goals in the first 24 hours.

BACKGROUND

The American College of Cardiology/American Heart Association (ACC/AHA) 2017 guidance for the prevention, detection, evaluation, and management of high blood pressure in adults defines hypertension (HTN) as a systolic blood pressure (SBP) greater than 120 mm Hg and diastolic blood pressure (DBP) greater than 80 mm Hg. The prevalence of HTN worldwide is 30% to 45%, and a strong association between HTN and clinical morbidity and mortality, particularly cardiovascular, has been established.[1] Hypertensive crisis (HTN-C) is an acute complication of HTN defined as a severe increase in blood pressure to more than 180/120 mm Hg and can be broken further into 2 subcategories: hypertensive emergency (HTN-E) and hypertensive urgency (HTN-U) based on the presence or absence of end-organ damage, respectively.[2] HTN-E, if left untreated, is associated with greater than 79% 1-year mortality and a median survival of 10.4 months.[1] Given the multitude of pharmacologic

[a] Baptist Memorial Hospital – Memphis, 6019 Walnut Grove Drive, Memphis, TN 38120, USA; [b] University of Tennessee Health Science Center College of Pharmacy, 881 Madison Avenue, Memphis, TN 38163, USA
* Corresponding author.
E-mail address: jfarrar7@uthsc.edu

Physician Assist Clin 8 (2023) 293–303
https://doi.org/10.1016/j.cpha.2022.10.009
physicianassistant.theclinics.com

agents available for the treatment of HTN-C, clinicians should understand individual-specific and disease-specific recommendations to optimize patient outcomes. The purpose of this review is to discuss pharmacotherapeutic interventions for hypertensive crises.

PATHOPHYSIOLOGY

The pathophysiology of HTN-C has not been fully elucidated; however, there are multiple physiologic processes that have been suggested. The heterogeneous causes of HTN allow for a variety of pharmacotherapeutic options targeting implicated mechanisms such as overactivation of the renin-angiotensin-aldosterone system, endothelial dysfunction, dysregulated nitric oxide secretion, and hyperinflammation.[2,3] In HTN-E, end-organ damage typically involves cardiovascular, cerebrovascular, pulmonary, and kidney organ systems and can manifest in a variety of ways including encephalopathy, intracerebral hemorrhage (ICH), acute ischemic stroke, myocardial infarction, pulmonary edema, aortic dissection, acute kidney injury, or eclampsia, to name a few. Patients presenting with HTN-U have similarly elevated blood pressure values to HTN-E (>180/120 mm Hg) but do not demonstrate any of the associated end-organ damage. However, these patients are at risk of developing organ damage and converting to HTN-E. Patients presenting with HTN-C necessitate emergency evaluation and intervention to prevent the development or worsening of end-organ damage.[1–3]

CLINICAL PRESENTATION AND TREATMENT GOALS

Clinical presentation of HTN-C varies but often involves nonspecific symptoms such as headache, dizziness, or angina. Given the high risk for morbidity and mortality if HTN-C is left untreated, patients presenting with elevated blood pressure should quickly undergo thorough evaluation. Potential causes of HTN and identification of end-organ damage can be determined through physical examination, urinalysis, and laboratory work including a complete blood count, basic metabolic panel, troponin, and b-type natriuretic peptide. There is a paucity of randomized trials evaluating optimal treatment of HTN-C; however, expert opinion suggests treatment stratified by presence (HTN-E) or absence (HTN-U) of end-organ damage.[1]

In patients presenting with HTN-E, clinicians should aim to lower blood pressure 20% to 25% in the first hour, using short-acting parenteral agents (**Table 1**), unless otherwise guided by end-organ disease (**Table 2**). Assuming the patient remains hemodynamically stable, blood pressure should then be reduced to 160/100 mm Hg during the next 2 to 6 hours, then cautiously to normal (<120/80 mm Hg) during the next 24 to 48 hours.[1,2] Certain clinical scenarios warrant special consideration of the underlying pathophysiology of the heterogenous cause of the HTN-E.

Because progressive damage is not present in HTN-U, initial blood pressure lowering can be accomplished with oral medications over 24 hours without the need for a more acute decrease or parenteral agents. Outpatient blood pressure goals outlined by the 2017 ACC/AHA Guidelines may be targeted.[1]

PHARMACOLOGIC MANAGEMENT: HYPERTENSIVE EMERGENCY

Stroke

The cerebral vascular system has a unique ability to maintain normotension through cerebral autoregulation. This comes from the ability of the cerebral vasculature to adapt to hypoperfusion or hyperperfusion through vasoconstriction or dilation. This

Table 1
Parental agents for hypertensive emergency[1]

Drug	Mechanism	Onset of Action	Dosing	Clinical Pearls
Nicardipine	Calcium channel blocker (dihydropyridine)	2–5 min	CIVI 5–15 mg/h *Titrate by 2.5 mg/h every 5 min; max 15 mg/h*	• Preferred in ischemic/hemorrhagic stroke • Risk of reflex tachycardia • Large volumes (up to 75 mL/h of NS)
Clevidipine	Calcium channel blocker (dihydropyridine)	2–4 min	CIVI 1–6 mg/h *Titrate by 1–2 mg/h every 90 s; max 32 mg/h*	• Preferred in ischemic/hemorrhagic stroke • Prepared in lipid emulsion (2 kcal/mL) • Avoid in patients allergic to soy or egg
Labetalol	α-1 adrenergic (selective) and β-adrenergic (nonselective) blocker	5 min	IV bolus 10–20 mg *Repeat escalating doses of 20–80 mg every 5–10 min PRN*	• Preferred in ischemic/hemorrhagic stroke, myocardial infarction, aortic dissection, and pregnant patients • Contraindicated in ADHF
Esmolol	Beta-blocker (cardioselective)	2–10 min	CIVI 25–300 mcg/kg/min *Titrate by 25 mcg/kg/min every 3–5 min; max 300 mcg/kg/min*	• Preferred in aortic dissection • Contraindicated in ADHF • Metabolism is organ independent (hydrolyzed by plasma esterases)
Enalaprilat	ACE inhibitor	15 min	IV bolus 1.25 mg every 6 h *Titrate no more than every 12 h; max 5 mg every 6 h*	• Contraindicated in pregnancy • Preferred in ADHF • Caution in renal dysfunction
Nitroprusside	Nitrate (vasodilator)	2 min	CIVI 0.25–10 mcg/kg/min *Titrate by 0.1–0.2 mcg/kg/min every 5 min*	• Avoid in ICP elevation, myocardial infarct (coronary steal) • Use in liver failure and renal failure can lead to cyanide toxicity • Toxicity with prolonged infusions (>72 h) or high doses (>3 mcg/kg/min)
Nitroglycerin	Nitrate (veno > arterial vasodilator)	<1 min	CIVI 5–200 mcg/min *Titrate by 5–25 mcg/kg/min every 5–10 min*	• Preferred in coronary ischemia, ADHF, pulmonary edema

(*continued on next page*)

Table 1
(*continued*)

Drug	Mechanism	Onset of Action	Dosing	Clinical Pearls
				• Tachyphylaxis occurs rapidly and requires uptitration • Contraindicated in patients using PDE-5 inhibitors (eg, sildenafil)
Fenoldapam	Peripheral D-1 receptor agonist	10 min	CIVI 0.03–1.6 mcg/kg/min *Titrate by 0.05–1 mcg/kg/min every 15 min*	• Risk of reflex tachycardia • Can cause ICP elevation, hypokalemia, and flushing
Hydralazine	Direct arterial vasodilator	10 min	IV bolus 10–20 mg every 30 min as needed	• Preferred in pregnancy • Risk of reflex tachycardia • Side effects: headaches, lupus-like syndromes, potent arterial vasodilation (hypotension)
Phentolamine	Pure α-adrenergic antagonist	1–2 min	IV bolus 1–5 mg as needed (Max 15 mg)	• Use in catecholamine-induced HTN-E (pheochromocytoma)

Abbreviations: ADHF, acute decompensated heart failure; CIVI, continuous intravenous infusion; HTN-E, hypertensive emergency; ICP, intracranial pressure; PRN, as needed.

Table 2
Blood pressure goals in end-organ damage[1,7]

End-Organ Damage	Preferred Agent	Hour 1 BP Reduction Goal	Hour 2–72 h BP Reduction Goal
ICH	• Nicardipine • Clevidipine • Labetalol	SBP 140 mm Hg (goal 130–150 mm Hg)	SBP 130–150 mm Hg
Ischemic stroke	• Nicardipine • Clevidipine • Labetalol	<180/105 mm Hg (TPA) <220/120 mm Hg (no TPA)	<180/105 mm Hg for 24 h (TPA) <220/120 mm Hg (no TPA)
Encephalopathy	• Nicardipine • Labetalol	SBP reduced by 25%	<160/100 mm Hg within 6 h and to normal in 24–48 h
Acute coronary syndrome	• Esmolol • Labetalol • Nicardipine • Nitroglycerin	SBP reduced by 25%	<160/100 mm Hg within 6 h and to normal in 24–48 h
Acute aortic dissection	• Esmolol • Labetalol	SBP <120 mm Hg	SBP <120 mm Hg
Acute heart failure	• Clevidipine • Nitroglycerin • Enalaprilat	SBP reduced by 25%	<160/100 mm Hg within 6 h and to normal in 24–48 h
Pulmonary edema	• Clevidipine • Nitroglycerin • Nitroprusside	SBP reduced by 25%	<160/100 mm Hg within 6 h and to normal in 24–48 h
Preeclampsia/ eclampsia	• Hydralazine • Labetalol • Nicardipine	SBP <140 mm Hg	SBP <140 mm Hg
Sympathetic crisis	• Clevidipine • Nicardipine • Phentolamine	SBP <140 mm Hg	SBP <140 mm Hg
Acute kidney injury	• Clevidipine • Fenoldopam • Nicardipine	SBP reduced by 25%	<160/100 mm Hg within 6 h and to normal in 24–48 h

Abbreviations: ICH, intracerebral hemorrhage; SBP, systolic blood pressure; TPA, tissue plasminogen activator.

intrinsic capacity, however, has physiologic limits, and the point at which the blood pressure exceeds the upper limit of autoregulatory capacity, cerebral tissue is at risk of hyperperfusion.[3,4] Hypertensive encephalopathy occurs when elevated intravascular pressure leads to leakage of intravascular fluid into cerebral tissue and increased intracranial pressure (ICP). Symptoms include headache, confusion, visual changes, nausea/vomiting, seizures, and coma. Clinicians should cautiously lower blood pressure by 25% in the first hour with easily titratable agents, such as nicardipine, clevidipine, or labetalol, given the risk of ischemic injury from cerebral tissue hypoperfusion if blood pressure is reduced too rapidly.[3,5] The presence of stroke, both ischemic and hemorrhagic, should be considered given the lack of cerebral autoregulatory capacity in these patients. The American Heart Association/American Stroke Association (AHA/ASA) guidelines recommend stratifying patients experiencing ischemic injury into 2 groups: those receiving thrombolysis and those who are not thrombolytic candidates. If a patient is receiving thrombolysis, blood pressure should be lowered to less than 185/110 mm Hg before the initiation of the IV thrombolytic and maintained less than 180/105 mm Hg for the subsequent 24 hours following administration. In those not receiving thrombolysis, blood pressure should only be treated when it exceeds 220/110 mm Hg in order to allow a normal autoregulatory response to maintain cerebral tissue perfusion. Patients with BP greater than 220/115 mm Hg should have BP lowered 15% in the first 24 hours. First-line agents include rapid-acting and titratable agents such as clevidipine and nicardipine with utilization of labetalol boluses as needed to achieve blood pressure control.[1,6] Patients developing ICH present a unique challenge given the negative consequences of both hypotension and HTN and the lack of heterogenous evidence in this population. The 2022 AHA/ASA Guidelines for Acute Management of ICH recommend acute lowering of SBP to target 140 mm Hg with a goal of maintaining a range of 130 mm Hg to 150 mm Hg. Acutely lowering presenting SBP greater than 150 mm Hg to less than 130 mm Hg was found to be harmful in this population. It is recommended to initiate antihypertensive treatment within 2 hours of ICH and reach target blood pressure within 1 hour. Rapidly titrated agents (nicardipine, clevidipine) should be used to ensure continuous smooth and sustained blood pressure control and to avoid large variability to improve functional outcomes.[7]

Aortic dissection

Uncontrolled HTN is one of the most modifiable risk factors in aortic dissection. Patients with acute aortic syndromes typically present with upper back or chest pain and shortness of breath necessitating chest radiograph or computed tomography scan to confirm diagnosis. First-line agents in this population include rapid-acting beta-blockers such as labetalol or esmolol to control both blood pressure and heart rate while maximizing myocardial oxygen supply and demand. Treatment aims specifically at decreasing the aortic pulsatile stress and minimizing further damage to the dissecting vessel. Second-line agents include nicardipine, nitroprusside, and clevidipine.[8]

Eclampsia and preeclampsia

Eclampsia and preeclampsia are life-threatening conditions that can develop in women 20 weeks after gestation. The American College of Obstetricians and Gynecologist (ACOG) defines preeclampsia as a single occasion of SBP 160 mm Hg or greater or DBP 110 mm Hg or greater at any time, or SBP 140 mm Hg or greater or DBP 90 mm Hg or greater on 2 occasions 4 hours apart. Eclampsia is when a woman with preeclampsia develops new onset grand mal seizures. The 2017 ACOG guidance for treatment of eclampsia and preeclampsia recommend intravenous labetalol and hydralazine as first line to a goal SBP of less than 140 mm Hg in the first hour of treatment. However, hydralazine is a potent arterial vasodilator and should be used with caution given the unpredictable maternal hypotensive effect. Oral immediate-release nifedipine should only be used in scenarios where IV access is not an option. Enalaprilat is contraindicated in pregnancy and nitroprusside should be used with caution, given the risk of cyanide toxicity and potential ICP elevation.[9,10]

Pheochromocytoma

Pheochromocytoma is a rare condition caused by a catecholamine-secreting tumor that creates a hyperadrenergic state. Patients present with headache, anxiety, palpitations, diaphoresis, and sustained HTN despite traditional antihypertensive pharmacotherapy. Treatment includes alpha-blocking agents, such as phentolamine, to control catecholamine activation of the adrenergic system. Beta-blocking agents

Table 3
Common first-line oral agents for hypertensive urgency[1,15–25]

Drug	Mechanism	Time to Peak Onset	Initial Dosing
Captopril	ACE inhibitor	1–1.5 h	6.25–25 mg every 8–12 h
Enalapril		4–6 h	5–10 mg/d
Lisinopril		7 h	5–10 mg/d
Ramipril		1 h	2.5 mg/d
Losartan	ARB	1 h	25–50 mg/d
Telmisartan		1 h	20–40 mg/d
Valsartan		2–4 h	80–160 mg/d
Amlodipine	DHP CCB	6–12 h	5–10 mg/d
Nifedipine XL/ER		20 min	30–60 mg/d
Chlorthalidone	Thiazide diuretic	2–6 h	12.5–25 mg/d
Hydrochlorothiazide		4 h	12.5–25 mg/d

Abbreviations: CCB, calcium channel blocker; DHP, dihydropyridine.

may be added as supportive therapy; however, definitive treatment requires the surgical removal of the adrenal gland with the tumor.[11]

PHARMACOLOGIC MANAGEMENT: HYPERTENSIVE URGENCY

Of patients who present with HTN-C, approximately 75% present with HTN-U.[12] Initial blood pressure lowering can be accomplished with oral medications during a 24-hour period due to the absence of progressive organ damage. The 2017 ACC/AHA guidelines provide blood pressure goals to be achieved during a 24 to 48-hour period in HTN-U.[1]

Medication noncompliance or nonadherence, substance abuse, and other factors related to comorbidities (i.e., end-stage kidney disease requiring renal replacement therapy) are all common risk factors for HTN-U–related hospital admissions.[13,14] Therefore, treatment of HTN-U often constitutes reinitiation of outpatient medication regimens if nonadherence is the suspected primary cause. Common first-line oral antihypertensives including dihydropyridine calcium channel blockers, thiazide diuretics, angiotensin converting enzyme inhibitors, and angiotensin receptor blockers may be found in **Table 3**.[1]

Table 4
Common second-line oral agents for hypertensive urgency[1,3,26–36]

Drug	Mechanism	Time to Peak Onset	Dosing
Atenolol	Beta-blocker	2–4 h	25 mg every 12–24 h
Bisoprolol		2–4 h	2.5–5 mg/d
Carvedilol		1–2 h	6.25 mg every 12 h
Labetalol		2–4 h	100 mg every 8–12 h
Metoprolol		1–2 h	25–50 mg every 12–24 h
Doxazosin	Alpha-blocker	2–3 h	1 mg/d
Prazosin		2–4 h	1–2 mg/d
Terazosin		2–3 h	1 mg/d
Clonidine	$Alpha_2$ agonist	1–3 h	0.1 mg every 8–12 h
Methyldopa		3–6 h	250 mg every 8–12 h
Hydralazine	Direct vasodilator	1–2 h	10–25 mg every 6–8 h

Patients may present with HTN-U due to a lack of access to primary care physicians and subsequent lack of medication optimization at follow-up. Many pharmacotherapeutic agents may require multiple titrations to achieve optimal blood pressure control. Second-line antihypertensives may include beta-blockers, alpha-blockers, hydralazine, and clonidine for refractory disease (**Table 4**). Addition of one or more agents may be necessary to achieve blood pressure goals after admission for HTN-U.

SUMMARY

HTN-C can have multiple different presentations and degrees of severity, which require specific treatment goals and agents. HTN-E requires emergent but measured blood pressure lowering with faster acting pharmacologic agents due to the presence of end-organ damage. HTN-U poses the risk of progression to end-organ damage but the absence of actual damage allows for a longer timeframe to achieve blood pressure control and can typically be resolved with oral antihypertensives. Patient-specific and disease-specific factors should be considered when choosing pharmacotherapeutic agents for the treatment of HTN-C.

EXAMPLE CASES AND ASSESSMENTS

Case 1:

CR is a 57-year-old woman with a medical history of systolic heart failure (left ventricular ejection fraction 25%), HTN, insulin-dependent diabetes, tobacco abuse, and gout. She presented to the emergency department with altered mental status and generalized weakness for the past 3 days after running out of her medications. Her initial vital assessment revealed a SBP/DBP of 220/130mm Hg (mean arterial pressure 160 mm Hg), HR 100 and Temp 97.5. Electrocardiogram showed normal sinus rhythm. Her laboratory work was as follows:

Na: 140 mEq/L | Cl: 110 mEq/L | K: 5.6 mmol/L | Scr: 4.2 mg/dL | CO2: 22 mEq/L
(Baseline serum creatinine 0.7 mg/dL)

Which is the most appropriate management for CR?

1. Use esmolol to achieve a goal of 25% reduction in MAP during the first 60 minutes
2. Use clevidipine to achieve a goal of 25% reduction in MAP during the first 60 minutes
3. Restart home oral antihypertensive agents to reduce MAP to goal in the first 24 hours
4. Use enalaprilat to achieve a goal of 50% reduction in MAP during the first 60 minutes.

Explanation

The correct answer is #2. This patient is presenting with HTN-E with a BP greater than 180/120 mm Hg and laboratory signs of acute kidney injury. She should have her BP lowered 20% to 25% in the first 60 minutes with a rapid acting parenteral agent. Esmolol is not preferred in patients with heart failure given the negative inotropic effects from the cardioselective beta antagonism. Enalaprilat is a preferred agent in heart failure; however, given her acute kidney failure, it should be used with caution. Clevidipine is a rapid-acting parenteral agent that is preferred in this patient with both chronic systolic heart failure and acute kidney injury. Restarting home oral antihypertensive agents to lower blood pressure to goal during the next 24 hours would be an option if she was presenting with HTN-U and no signs of end-organ damage.

Case 2:

RL is a 46-year-old woman with a past medical history of type 2 diabetes, HTN, and stage 2 chronic kidney disease presenting to the emergency department with signs and symptoms consistent with diabetic ketoacidosis. Vital signs are collected: blood pressure, 189/98 mm Hg; heart rate, 64 beats per minute; respiratory rate, 32 breaths per minute; and oxygen saturation, 93%. RL admits to running out of her home medications last week, including insulin glargine 25 units daily, dapagliflozin 10 mg daily, and lisinopril 20 mg daily.

Which of the following is the most appropriate intervention to treat RL's HTN-U?

1. Administer labetalol 10 mg IV once to decrease SBP to less than 160 mm Hg
2. Initiate chlorthalidone 25 mg daily to decrease blood pressure to less than 180/100 mm Hg within 24 hours
3. Reinitiate lisinopril 20 mg PO daily to decrease blood pressure to outpatient goal within 48 hours
4. Initiate amlodipine 10 mg PO daily to decrease blood pressure to outpatient goal within 24 hours

Explanation

The correct answer is #3. This patient should be diagnosed with an HTN-U—her SBP is greater than 180 mm Hg but she is not yet experiencing any signs of organ damage. She has not taken her home medications in about a week, indicating that the likely cause of her HTN-U is nonadherence. The most appropriate intervention would be to reinitiate her home antihypertensive (lisinopril) and monitor blood pressure for return to outpatient goals within 24 to 48 hours. This patient does not warrant IV therapy at this time due to the lack of organ damage associated with her HTN. If this patient remained uncontrolled after reinitiation of her home regimen, the addition of chlorthalidone or amlodipine (2 first-line oral agents for the treatment of HTN) may be appropriate to achieve blood pressure goals.

CLINICS CARE POINTS

- HTN-E involves end-organ damage, whereas HTN-U does not.
- Intravenous antihypertensive agents should be used for HTN-E, and oral antihypertensives should be used for HTN-U.
- Intravenous agents and blood pressure goals may be selected based on organ-specific and disease-specific considerations in HTN-E.
- Oral agents (often existing home medications) may be used to lower blood pressure in HTN-U.

DISCLOSURE

The authors have nothing to disclose.

REFERENCES

1. Whelton PK, Carey RM, Aronow WS, et al. 2017 ACC/AHA/AAPA/ABC/ACPM/AGS/APhA/ASH/ASPC/NMA/PCNa guideline for the prevention, detection, evaluation, and management of high blood pressure in adults: a report of the American

College of Cardiology/American Heart Association Task Force on Clinical Practice Guidelines. Hypertension 2018;71(6):e13–115.

2. Ipek E, Oktay AA, Krim SR. Hypertensive crisis: an update on clinical approach and management. Curr Opin Cardiol 2017;32:397–406.
3. Brathwaite L, Reif M. Hypertensive Emergencies: A Review of Common Presentations and Treatment Options. Cardiol Clin 2019;37:275–86.
4. Armstead WM. Cerebral Blood Flow Autoregulation and Dysautoregulation. Anesthesiol Clin 2016;34(3):465–77.
5. Manning L, Robinson TG, Anderson CS. Control of blood pressure in hypertensive neurological emergencies. Curr Hypertens Rep 2014;16(6):436.
6. Powers WJ, Rabinstein AA, Ackerson T, et al. Guidelines for the early management of patients with acute ischemic stroke: a guideline for healthcare professionals from the America heart association/American stroke association. Stroke 2018;49(3):e46–110.
7. Greenberg SM, Ziai WC, Cordonnier C, et al. Guideline for the Management of Patients With Spontaneous Intracerebral Hemorrhage: A Guideline From the American Heart Association/American Stroke Association. Stroke 2022;53:00.
8. Gupta PK, Gupta H, Khonynezhad A. Hypertensive Emergency in Aortic Dissection and Thoracic Aortic Aneursym- A Review of Management. Pharmaceuticals 2009;2(3):66–76.
9. American College of Obstetrics and gynecolosist Task Force on Hypertension in Pregnancy. Hypertension in pregnancy. Report of the American College of Obstetricians and Gynecologists' Task Force on Hypertension in Pregnancy. Obstet Gynecol 2013;122(5):1122–31.
10. Vadhera RB, Simon M. Hypertensive Emergencies in Pregnancy. Clin Obstet Gynecol 2014;57(4):797–805.
11. Sbardella E, Grossman AB. Pheochromocytoma: An approach to diagnosis. Best Pract Res Clin Endocrinol Metab 2020;34(2):101346.
12. Pinna G, Pascale C, Fornengo P, et al. Hospital admissions for hypertensive crisis in the emergency departments: a large multicenter Italian study. PLoS One 2014;9:1–6.
13. Gore JM, Peterson E, Amin A, et al. Predictors of 90-day readmission among patients with acute severe hypertension. The cross-sectional observational Studying the Treatment of Acute hyperTension (STAT) study. Am Heart J 2010;160:521–7.
14. Saguner AM, Du€r S, Perrig M, et al. Risk factors promoting hypertensive crises: evidence from a longitudinal study. Am J Hypertens 2010;23:775–80.
15. Captopril. Lexi-Drugs. Lexicomp. Wolters Kluwer, Inc. Riverwoods, IL. Available at: http://online.lexi.com. Accessed April 12, 2022.
16. Enalapril. Lexi-Drugs. Lexicomp. Wolters Kluwer, Inc. Riverwoods, IL. Available at: http://online.lexi.com. Accessed April 12, 2022.
17. Lisinopril. Lexi-Drugs. Lexicomp. Wolters Kluwer, Inc. Riverwoods, IL. Available at: http://online.lexi.com. Accessed April 12, 2022.
18. Ramipiril. Lexi-Drugs. Lexicomp. Wolters Kluwer, Inc. Riverwoods, IL. Available at: http://online.lexi.com. Accessed April 12, 2022.
19. Losartan. Lexi-Drugs. Lexicomp. Wolters Kluwer, Inc. Riverwoods, IL. Available at: http://online.lexi.com. Accessed April 12, 2022.
20. Telmisartan. Lexi-Drugs. Lexicomp. Wolters Kluwer, Inc. Riverwoods, IL. Available at: http://online.lexi.com. Accessed April 12, 2022.
21. Valsartan. Lexi-Drugs. Lexicomp. Wolters Kluwer, Inc. Riverwoods, IL. Available at: http://online.lexi.com. Accessed April 12, 2022.

22. Amlodipine. Lexi-Drugs. Lexicomp. Wolters Kluwer, Inc. Riverwoods, IL. Available at: http://online.lexi.com. Accessed April 12, 2022.
23. Nifedipine. Lexi-Drugs. Lexicomp. Wolters Kluwer, Inc. Riverwoods, IL. Available at: http://online.lexi.com. Accessed April 12, 2022.
24. Chlorthalidone. Lexi-Drugs. Lexicomp. Wolters Kluwer, Inc. Riverwoods, IL. Available at: http://online.lexi.com. Accessed April 12, 2022.
25. Hydrochlorothiazide. Lexi-Drugs. Lexicomp. Wolters Kluwer, Inc. Riverwoods, IL. Available at: http://online.lexi.com. Accessed April 12, 2022.
26. Atenolol. Lexi-Drugs. Lexicomp. Wolters Kluwer, Inc. Riverwoods, IL. Available at: http://online.lexi.com. Accessed April 12, 2022.
27. Bisoprolol. Lexi-Drugs. Lexicomp. Wolters Kluwer, Inc. Riverwoods, IL. Available at: http://online.lexi.com. Accessed April 12, 2022.
28. Carvedilol. Lexi-Drugs. Lexicomp. Wolters Kluwer, Inc. Riverwoods, IL. Available at: http://online.lexi.com. Accessed April 12, 2022.
29. Labetalol. Lexi-Drugs. Lexicomp. Wolters Kluwer, Inc. Riverwoods, IL. Available at: http://online.lexi.com. Accessed April 12, 2022.
30. Metoprolol. Lexi-Drugs. Lexicomp. Wolters Kluwer, Inc. Riverwoods, IL. Available at: http://online.lexi.com. Accessed April 12, 2022.
31. Doxazosin. Lexi-Drugs. Lexicomp. Wolters Kluwer, Inc. Riverwoods, IL. Available at: http://online.lexi.com. Accessed April 12, 2022.
32. Prazosin. Lexi-Drugs. Lexicomp. Wolters Kluwer, Inc. Riverwoods, IL. Available at: http://online.lexi.com. Accessed April 12, 2022.
33. Terazosin. Lexi-Drugs. Lexicomp. Wolters Kluwer, Inc. Riverwoods, IL. Available at: http://online.lexi.com. Accessed April 12, 2022.
34. Clonidine. Lexi-Drugs. Lexicomp. Wolters Kluwer, Inc. Riverwoods, IL. Available at: http://online.lexi.com. Accessed April 12, 2022.
35. Methyldopa. Lexi-Drugs. Lexicomp. Wolters Kluwer, Inc. Riverwoods, IL. Available at: http://online.lexi.com. Accessed April 12, 2022.
36. Hydralazine. Lexi-Drugs. Lexicomp. Wolters Kluwer, Inc. Riverwoods, IL. Available at: http://online.lexi.com. Accessed April 12, 2022.

Best Practices in Medical Management of Chronic Hypertension

Rebecca Boyle, MSPA, PA-C[a,*], Lauren Remer, MSPA, PA-S[b]

KEYWORDS

• Hypertension • Blood pressure • Antihypertensive agents

KEY POINTS

When considering whether to initiate antihypertensive therapy, the following questions can be a helpful framework to guide medical management or need for further diagnostics:

- Does this patient have hypertension?
- Does this patient have an identifiable cause driving their hypertension?
- Should this patient be treated with antihypertensive medications?
- Are there compelling indications for this patient?
- Are there any medications that should be avoided?
- What is the target of treatment?

INTRODUCTION

This article provides a basic guide on the medical management of primary or "essential" hypertension in the nonpregnant adult in the outpatient setting. Evaluation and management of hypertensive emergencies (see chapter 6), hypertension in hospitalized patients, and hypertension due to an identifiable underlying cause ("secondary hypertension") are beyond the scope of this discussion.

The clinical relevance of hypertension cannot be understated. Hypertension is ubiquitous, present in nearly 1 of every 2 adults in the United States.[1] The disorder is likewise insidious, often referred to as "the silent killer." Despite the absence of overt symptoms, elevated blood pressure is the leading risk factor for stroke[2] and is considered a contributing cause of death in more than 500,000 US individuals annually.[1] Additional complications of uncontrolled hypertension include chronic kidney disease, retinopathy, and cardiomyopathy. The cost of hypertension extends beyond the physical, resulting in US medical expenditures of upward of $131 billion

[a] Inpatient Medicine, Stanford Healthcare, Palo Alto, CA, USA; [b] Inpatient Medicine, Stanford Health Care - ValleyCare, 5555 West Las Positas Boulevard, Pleasanton, CA 94588, USA
* Corresponding author. 300 Pasteur Dr, Stanford, CA 94305.
E-mail address: RBoyle@stanfordhealthcare.org

Physician Assist Clin 8 (2023) 305–317
https://doi.org/10.1016/j.cpha.2022.10.014
physicianassistant.theclinics.com

annually.[1] Unfortunately, only 1 in 4 individuals with hypertension has their blood pressure under control.[1] These observations highlight the opportunity for improvements in blood pressure management to translate to significant reductions in mortality and morbidity.

When considering whether to initiate antihypertensive therapy, the following questions can be a helpful framework to guide medical management or need for further diagnostics:

1. Does this patient have hypertension?
2. Does this patient have an identifiable cause driving their hypertension (secondary hypertension)?
3. Should this patient be treated with antihypertensive medications?
4. Are there compelling indications for this patient to be on specific medications?
5. Are there any medications that should be avoided in this particular patient?
6. What is the target of treatment?

Does This Patient Have Hypertension?

For the purposes of this article, hypertension is defined as in the 2017 American College of Cardiology/American Heart Association (ACC/AHA) *High Blood Pressure Clinical Practice Guidelines*,[3] which considers normal adult blood pressure less than 120/80 mm Hg, elevated blood pressure 120 to 129/80 mm Hg, stage I hypertension 130 to 139/80 to 89 mm Hg, and stage II hypertension greater than or equal to 140/90 mm Hg. It should be recognized that not all major clinical practice guidelines agree on the definition of hypertension or the blood pressure target for treatment. For example, the 2020 International Society of Hypertension (ISH) Global Hypertension Practice Guidelines[4] consider normal blood pressure to be less than 130/less than 85 mm Hg, "high normal" blood pressure 130 to 139/85 to 89 mm Hg, and grade I hypertension to be 140 to 159/90 to 99 mm Hg. In light of data from the SPRINT & STEP blood pressure trials[5,6] demonstrating all-cause mortality and incidence of cardiovascular events, respectively, from lower blood pressure targets (systolic blood pressure [SBP] <120 in SPRINT and SBP target 110–130 mm Hg in STEP blood pressure), this article incorporates the stricter ACC/AHA definition of hypertension in order to alert clinicians to a wider range of patients who may benefit from antihypertensive therapy. Selection of blood pressure targets on treatment is addressed later.

Regardless of the blood pressure cutoff used to diagnose hypertension, it is widely accepted that the diagnosis is not made on a single reading.[4] The US Preventive Services Task Force gives a grade A recommendation to confirming the diagnosis of hypertension with "blood pressure measurements outside of the clinical setting."[2] Many medical offices do not have a workflow in place to dedicate the time and space recommended for accurate blood pressure measurement, in which a patient is placed in a quiet environment, allowed to relax for several minutes, and seated with back supported, feet flat on the floor and arm supported to rest at the level of the heart. The difference between nonstandardized blood pressure measurements and carefully obtained readings in clinical trials can be quite stark, with dramatic implications for therapy decisions. In one example, Drawz and colleagues compared patient blood pressures as measured as the mean of 3 readings taken in a quiet, unattended environment with blood pressures obtained on a single, nonstandardized reading from a routine office visit. In this study, blood pressures were found to vary by as much as 45 mm Hg in the same individual undergoing readings with the 2 different measurement techniques.[7] Clinicians are encouraged to review the recommended office blood pressure measurement protocol outlined in the 2020 ISH guidelines for measurement techniques to optimize accuracy. Factors such as full bladder, recent ingestion of food, or talking during measurements can affect the accuracy of blood pressure readings, placing patients at risk of inaccurately being labeled as hypertensive or normotensive. If office blood pressure readings are used, at least 2 measurements with 1 minute between readings should be taken on 2 to 3 separate visits to confirm diagnosis.[4,5]

Alternative means of diagnosing hypertension include ambulatory blood pressure monitoring, typically obtained over 24 hours by a device measuring blood pressure every 20 to 30 minutes or home blood pressure readings using a validated device. Ambulatory and home blood pressure monitoring are critical in uncovering cases of "white coat hypertension" (hypertensive blood pressure in clinical settings with normal out of office blood pressure) and "masked hypertension" (normal blood pressure in clinical settings with hypertensive out of office blood pressure), which would otherwise be missed on office blood pressure readings alone. In healthy individuals, blood pressures drop or "dip" during sleep; thus, if nocturnal blood pressures are used in diagnosis, there is a lower blood pressure threshold for diagnosing hypertension. Failure of blood pressure dipping during sleep is associated with poor cardiovascular prognosis.[8] In patients undergoing ambulatory blood pressure, diagnostic thresholds for diagnosis of hypertension include a 24-hour average blood pressure greater than 125/75 mm Hg, daytime blood pressure greater than130/80 mm Hg, or night-time blood pressure greater than 110/65 mm Hg.[9] Patients performing home blood pressure monitoring can be directed to the Web site validatebp.org for a list of home blood pressure monitoring devices that have been verified by third parties for accuracy,[10] and they should be instructed on appropriate technique as outlined earlier for office measurements.[11]

Does This Patient Have an Identifiable Cause Driving Their Hypertension (Secondary Hypertension)?

Most, up to 95%, of all patients with hypertension have primary or "essential" hypertension, for which no specific underlying pathology can be identified.[2] A subset of patients, however, have secondary hypertension: elevated blood pressures driven by an identifiable cause. Identifying patients with secondary hypertension is clinically important, as treatment of the underlying cause can obviate long-term antihypertensive medication. Furthermore, allowing the driver of elevated blood pressures to go undiagnosed may place the patient at risk for long-term sequelae of the underlying disorder. One example can be seen in obstructive sleep apnea (OSA), a common cause of secondary hypertension. Treatment of sleep apnea with weight loss and/or continuous positive airway pressure can reduce the need for blood pressure medication, whereas treating blood pressure without addressing the underlying OSA leaves the patient vulnerable to the long-term risk of cardiac dysrhythmias, functional daytime impairment, and insulin resistance.[12]

The population of patients with resistant hypertension, defined as blood pressure that remains uncontrolled despite 3 medications including a diuretic or use of 4 or more antihypertensives for blood pressure control,[13] is particularly enriched with individuals with secondary hypertension. Up to 25% of patients with resistant hypertension have an underlying cause of secondary hypertension.[6] Resistant hypertension must be distinguished from "pseudoresistance" in which a patient is prescribed multiple blood pressure medications, but not adherent with treatment.

The medication strategies discussed later are intended to apply to patients with primary hypertension. However, clinicians should be aware of signs of potential secondary hypertension that would warrant further evaluation and diagnosis-specific treatment. Signs of select common causes of secondary hypertension are outlined in Appendix A available online.

Should This Patient Be Treated with Antihypertensive Medications?

All patients, regardless of blood pressure, should be encouraged to cultivate healthy lifestyle behavior patterns for both primary and secondary prevention of hypertension and their associated end-organ complications. The International Society of Hypertension recognizes lifestyle modification as the "first line of antihypertensive treatment."[4] Specific lifestyle modifications with evidenced-based blood pressure–lowering effect include weight loss, the DASH (Dietary Approach to Stop Hypertension) diet, sodium restriction, increased potassium intake in patients not at risk for hyperkalemia, physical activity, and moderation of alcohol consumption.[3,4,11] For some individuals, lifestyle modification may be sufficient to control hypertension. For those requiring pharmacologic therapy, lifestyle modification can enhance efficacy of antihypertensive treatment in addition to reducing overall risk of cardiovascular events.

ACC/AHA guidelines support a 3- to 6-month trial of lifestyle intervention before initiation of pharmacologic antihypertensive therapy in individuals with either (1) blood pressure less than 130/80 mm Hg or (2) blood pressure 130 to 139/80 to 89 mm Hg who do not have clinical atherosclerotic cardiovascular disease (ASCVD) and estimated 10-year cardiovascular disease risk less than 10%.[11] In contrast, individuals in any of the following 4 categories are advised to supplement lifestyle modification with medication[14]:

1. Blood pressure greater than or equal to 140/90 mm Hg
2. Blood pressure 130 to 139/80 to 89 mm Hg and clinical ASCVD
3. Blood pressure 130 to 139/80 to 89 mm Hg and 10-year risk of cardiovascular disease greater than or equal to 10%
4. All individuals not meeting criteria for up-front medication therapy who have persistently elevated blood pressure greater than 130/80 mm Hg despite 6 months of lifestyle intervention.

Similarly, the International Society of Hypertension uses blood pressure at time of diagnosis and the presence or absence of high-risk comorbidities to distinguish when a trial of lifestyle optimization is appropriate from situations in which immediate medical therapy is warranted.[4]

Are There Compelling Indications for This Patient to Be on Specific Medications?

The term "compelling indication" refers to a high-risk medical comorbidity (the "indication") with authoritative ("compelling") outcome data or clinical practice guidelines to support the use of a specific class of antihypertensive therapy. The benefits associated with these agents may be independent of blood pressure control. For example, the presence of proteinuria is typically considered a compelling indication for use of an angiotensin-converting enzyme inhibitor (ACEI) or angiotensin receptor blocker (ARB). This recommendation is based on several outcomes trials including the Reduction of Endpoints in NIDDM with the Angiotensin II Antagonist Losartan (RENAAL) trial, which demonstrated that in patients with diabetic kidney disease, the ARB losartan reduced risk of progression to end-stage renal disease independent of blood pressure lowering effect.[15]

Patients with compelling indications should be started on the antihypertensive drug classes associated with favorable long-term clinical outcomes before alternative first-line agents (**Table 1**). As the benefit of therapy in these high-risk populations may be independent of blood pressure control, the decision to start medical therapy for

Table 1
Select compelling indications and recommended antihypertensive therapy

Compelling Indication	ACEI/ARB	Diuretic	β-Blocker	Calcium Channel Blocker	Mineralocorticoid Receptor Antagonist
Systolic heart failure	Recommended	Recommended for patients requiring volume management	Recommended	Avoid	Recommended
Postmyocardial infarction	Recommended	—	Recommended	—	Recommended
Proteinuric chronic kidney disease	Recommended	—	—	—	—
Poststroke	Recommended	Recommended	—	—	—

patients with compelling indications should not be based on the algorithms used for initiating antihypertensive therapy in the general population. Instead, agents with proven benefit should be started by default if blood pressure and side-effect profile permit.

Are There Any Medications that Should Be Avoided in This Particular Patient?

Regardless of whether a patient has a compelling indication to be on a specific pharmacologic agent, according to the principle of "do no harm," clinicians must also consider whether there are contraindications or side effects of therapy that would potentially outweigh expected benefit. Hypotension is a risk universal to all agents used for blood pressure reduction and can be particularly catastrophic in certain populations such as those with osteoporosis or on anticoagulation. For individuals with heightened risk of poor outcomes from hypotension, consider starting on low doses of a single agent, exercising a more liberal blood pressure target of therapy, and instituting more frequent clinical monitoring. Common and potential treatment-limiting side effects of the select blood pressure medications reviewed in this article are listed under the respective class of agents discussed later.

First-Line Agents

Consider starting with a combination pill or low-to-moderate doses of multiple first-line agents from 2 different classes. This practice is recommended by the 2020 ISH guidelines that outline ideal "Step One" therapy as a single pill combination of ACEI or ARB and dihydropyridine calcium channel blocker.[4] Recently the QUARTET trial demonstrated that patients randomized to receive a single "quadpill" containing a fixed dose of 4 distinct antihypertensive agents achieved and maintained better blood pressure control than patients assigned to start with monotherapy with subsequent upward titration.[16] The therapeutic benefit of upfront poly-therapy may stem from possible synergistic mechanisms of action of different medication classes as well as the potential to reduce clinician tendency toward therapeutic inertia. The relationship between antihypertensive dose and degree of blood pressure lowering is nonlinear. After a certain dosage threshold is reached, there is minimal additional antihypertensive benefit from dose escalation. Low-to-moderate dosing of multiple agents can allow patients to obtain the blood pressure benefit of being on therapy with reduced risk of adverse effect of being on high doses of any one agent.

Thiazides and thiazide-like agents

Common examples. *Chlorthalidone, hydrochlorothiazide, indapamide, metolazone*

Populations that may uniquely benefit

- "Salt-sensitive" patients
- Low-renin hypertension
- Hypercalciuria
- Poststroke
- Calcineurin inhibitor–mediated hypertension

Mechanism of action. Thiazides block the sodium-chloride symporter in the distal tubule of the kidneys, leading to enhanced excretion of sodium and diuretic effect. In the setting of stable sodium intake, the natriuretic and diuretic effect leads to short-term blood pressure reduction until the kidney is able to compensate and achieve a new steady state of sodium and water balance. Long-term antihypertensive benefit is speculated to be due to vasodilation by vascular potassium channel activation.[17]

Side effects potentially limiting therapeutic use

- Hyponatremia
- Hypokalemia
- Hypomagnesemia
- Hyperuricemia
- Polyuria (risk of polyuria can be largely reduced by avoiding high salt loads and use of longer-acting thiazide-like agents)

Notable mention. Chlorthalidone, a longer-acting thiazide-like agent, can be dosed as infrequently as 3 times weekly and retains antihypertensive efficacy even in advanced stages of chronic kidney disease (CKD).[18]

Angiotensin-converting enzyme inhibitors and angiotensin-2-receptor blockers
Common examples. *Lisinopril, captopril, enalapril, ramipril, losartan, olmesartan, valsartan, telmisartan, azilsartan, irbesartan*.

Populations that may uniquely benefit

- High-renin hypertension
- Proteinuria
- Poststroke
- Heart failure with reduced ejection fraction
- Post–myocardial infarction (MI)

Mechanism of action. ACEI and ARB decrease blood pressure through direct action on the renin-angiotensin-aldosterone system. ACEI inhibit the ACE that converts angiotensin I to angiotensin II. ARB blocks the binding of angiotensin II to its receptor. These actions produce similar effects through the prevention of arteriole vasoconstriction and aldosterone release, which dilates blood vessels and decreases sodium and water reabsorption in the distal tubule of the nephron, respectively.

Side effects potentially limiting therapeutic use

- Cough (ACEI specific)
- Angioedema
- Hyperkalemia (can now be mitigated by potassium binders, which is beyond the scope of this article)
- Pancreatitis
- Heightened risk of acute kidney injury during situations of reduced renal perfusion (poor oral intake, hypotension, renal artery stenosis) or concomitant use of nonsteroidal antiinflammatory agents

Notable mention. Azilsartan is recognized as the longest acting and most potent ARB.[6] Overall, use of ARBs is favored over ACEI due to less risk of cough, angioedema, and pancreatitis.[19]

Dihydropyridine and nondihydropyridine calcium channel blockers
Common examples. *Amlodipine, felodipine, nifedipine (DHP calcium channel blockers [CCB]) verapamil, diltiazem (non-DHP CCB)*

Populations that may uniquely benefit

- Low-renin hypertension
- After kidney transplant
- Raynaud phenomenon

Mechanism of action. Non-DHP CCB cause vasodilation of coronary and peripheral arteries and decrease cardiac contractility through blocking voltage-gated calcium channels in both cardiac and vascular muscle and are used primarily in treating tachydysrhythmias. DHP CCB block voltage-gated calcium changes in the vascular smooth muscle, resulting in vasodilation.

Side effects potentially limiting therapeutic use of dihydropyridine calcium channel blockers

- Peripheral edema (can be mitigated by dose reduction or concomitant use of ACEI or ARB; not typically responsive to diuretics)
- Constipation
- Flushing

Notable mention. Amlodipine and felodipine are the only 2 DHP CCB considered safe in patients with reduced systolic function.[20]

Second- and Third-Line Agents

If starting with a single agent, in the absence of compelling indications, second- and third-line therapy should consist of adding agents from each of the 3 "first-line" medication classes and optimizing doses. In particular, optimizing dose of the thiazide or thiazide-like agent, with strong consideration of use of chlorthalidone, may obviate addition of a fourth agent.

Fourth-Line Agents

For patients without compelling indications for β-blocker therapy, mineralocorticoid receptor antagonists (MRAs) are generally favored over β-blockers or α-blockers as fourth-line therapy for resistant hypertension given data showing increased efficacy of MRAs in lowering blood pressure.[21]

Mineralocorticoid receptor antagonists

Common examples. *Spironolactone, eplerenone.*

Populations that may uniquely benefit. Resistant hypertension, low-renin hypertension, patients desiring antiandrogen therapy (spironolactone).

- Heart failure with reduced ejection fraction, hyperaldosteronism, OSA.[22]

Mechanism of action. MRA competitively bind to nuclear aldosterone receptor sites in the distal renal tubules, resulting in decreased production of sodium channels, thereby impairing the ability to reabsorb sodium. Full antihypertensive effects from active metabolites of MRAs may take days to weeks to manifest.

Side effects potentially limiting therapeutic use

- Hyperkalemia
- Gynecomastia (spironolactone-specific)
- Menstrual irregularities (spironolactone-specific)

Notable mention. Eplerenone or non-MRA potassium sparing diuretics are favored over spironolactone in patients identifying as male given spironolactone's antiandrogen side effects.

Beta-adrenergic antagonists (β-blockers)

Common examples. *Carvedilol, metoprolol, bisoprolol, atenolol, nebivolol, labetalol.*

Populations that may uniquely benefit

- High-renin hypertension
- Post-MI

- Reduced systolic function
- Tachyarrhythmia

Mechanism of action. β-blockers act on the sympathetic nervous system. Its antihypertensive effects are primarily due to the blockade of β1 receptors on the heart and on the kidney. β1 blockade on the heart decreases chronotropy and inotropy, which decreases heart rate and contractility. β1 receptor blockers also act on the renin-angiotensin-aldosterone system by blocking β1 receptors on the smooth muscle cells of the juxtaglomerular apparatus of the kidney to decrease its renin release. Nonselective β-blockers block both β1 receptors as well as β2 adrenergic receptors found in airway smooth muscle cells.

Side effects potentially limiting therapeutic use

- Bradycardia
- Fatigue
- Depression
- Exacerbation of reactive airway disease (nonselective β-blockers)
- Erectile dysfunction

Notable mention. Nebivolol is a β-blocker with nitric oxide–mediated vasodilatory properties that may be more potent and carry fewer side effects than other agents in this class.[23] Evidence-based β-blockers for patients with reduced systolic function include bisoprolol, carvedilol, and metoprolol succinate.

Alpha-receptor antagonists

Common examples. *Doxazosin, prazosin, terazosin.*

Populations that may uniquely benefit

- Patients with blood pressure hyperplasia

Mechanism of action. Alpha-receptor antagonists modulate the sympathetic nervous system by blocking α1-adrenoreceptors in the peripheral vascular muscle, inhibiting vasoconstriction. Because of the vasodilation of both venous and arterioles, there is a decrease in total peripheral resistance and blood pressure.

Side effects potentially limiting therapeutic use

- First-dose hypotension
- Reflex tachycardia
- Floppy iris syndrome

Other agents. Use of antihypertensive agents beyond those included in traditional first through fourth-line drug classes should typically be limited to special circumstances. **Table 2** gives information on these other agents and when they could be considered. As noted earlier, the presence of resistant hypertension should raise the question of suboptimal medication compliance or secondary hypertension.

DISCUSSION: WHAT IS THE TARGET OF TREATMENT?

There is a lack of consensus among major clinical practice guidelines as to the optimal blood pressure target for patients with hypertension. Proponents of more intensive blood pressure control to a goal of systolic blood pressure less than 120 mm Hg often cite results of the SPRINT trial, which found a significant reduction in a composite outcome of cardiovascular disease events as well as reduction in all-cause mortality for patients in the intensive blood pressure control arm.[5] More support for lower blood

Table 2
Additional antihypertensive agents

Drug Class	Available Drugs	Clinical Scenarios for Use	ADRs
Loop diuretics	Furosemide, bumetanide, torsemide	Volume overload, especially in patients with heart failure or advanced CKD	Electrolyte abnormalities Acute kidney injury from dehydration
Alpha-2 receptor agonists	Clonidine	Patch for patients with adherence issues or swallowing issues	Vivid dreams Tachycardia
Potassium-sparing diuretics	Amiloride, triamterene	Liddle syndrome, syndromes of apparent mineralocorticoid excess	Hyperkalemia

pressure targets comes from the STEP Study Group, which conducted a trial demonstrating lower incidence of cardiovascular events among older adults (age 60–80 years) treated to a systolic blood pressure goal of 110 to 130 mm Hg as compared with those held to a more liberal systolic blood pressure target of 130 to 150 mm Hg.[6] Important considerations to the interpretation of these findings include the trials' methodology as well as inclusion and exclusion criteria. The SPRINT trial notably measured blood pressure as a mean of 3 unobserved blood pressure readings obtained via automated devices after patients were allowed 5 minutes of rest. This standardized technique is not widely used in routine clinical practice and, as noted earlier, was later shown to yield blood pressure readings sometimes widely variable from nonstandardized blood pressure readings obtained in the same patient.[7] The SPRINT trial's generalizability has also been challenged in its exclusion of diabetics as well as individuals with standing systolic blood pressures less than or equal to 110 mm Hg, potentially limiting applicability of more intensive blood pressure targets to these patient populations.

An example of contrasting blood pressure targets can be seen in comparison of the 2021 Kidney Disease Improving Global Outcomes (KDIGO) and the 2017 ACC/AHA blood pressure guidelines. KDIGO guidelines embrace an SPRINT-based systolic blood pressure target of less than 120 mm Hg for adults with CKD, with the caveat that obtaining standardized, accurate blood pressure readings is "crucial" and "integral" to holding patients accountable to this target.[24] Conversely, ACC/AHA guidelines set a more liberal blood pressure target of less than 130/80 mm Hg because that use of ideal blood pressure measurement technique such as in SPRINT is unfortunately not common practice.[11]

The lack of guideline consensus provides an opportunity for individualization of patient goals for antihypertensive therapy. Indeed, Itoga and colleagues found that different blood pressure targets may be appropriate for individuals with different risks of specific cardiovascular events, with blood pressure 140 to 155/70 to 80 mm Hg associated with lowest hazard ratio for all-cause mortality, blood pressure 110 to 120/85 to 90 mm Hg associated with the lowest hazard ratio for MI, and blood pressure 125 to 135/70 to 75 mm Hg associated with the lowest hazard ratio for heart failure and a linear relationship between systolic blood pressure and risk of stroke.[25] Elevated estimated cardiovascular risk as well as markers of hypertension-mediated organ damage, such as left ventricular hypertrophy, albuminuria, or retinopathy, may be signs that an individual stands to benefit from more intensive blood pressure control. However, there is a need for ongoing reassessment to ensure the risk/benefit ratio of medical management favors the patient. Outside factors influencing both blood pressure and a patient's predisposition to medication side effects may evolve over time. For example, significant weight loss or treatment of OSA may reduce or eliminate a patient's need to remain on antihypertensive drug therapy. Alternatively, patients may require periodic uptitration of their blood pressure regimen or change of antihypertensive medication class. With age, individuals may become increasingly salt sensitive, thus the use of a thiazide-like diuretic may become comparatively more effective over time. However, with age, individuals may also be more prone to the side effects of thiazide-like agents such as hyponatremia and orthostatic hypotension, highlighting the importance of regular clinical evaluation to ensure blood pressure remains controlled on a regimen the patient tolerates. When considering patients for deescalation of antihypertensive therapy, prioritize continuing agents for compelling indications, given favorable long-term outcomes associated with these agents.

SUMMARY

Although many algorithms exist to guide clinicians on blood pressure management, it is important to grasp the patient-specific factors that modify an individual's estimated clinical benefit from targeting lower blood pressures, as well as a patient's ability to tolerate commonly used antihypertensive agents. Firmly establishing the diagnosis of hypertension and exclusion of potential causes of secondary hypertension is essential in ensuring the appropriate initial prescription of blood pressure–lowering agents. Identifying patient populations with compelling indications for specific classes of antihypertensives can help prioritize agents with proven clinical benefit. Finally, understanding the basic physiologic mechanisms of first- and second-line agents can facilitate the selection of medications with the greatest risk/benefit ratio. Patients with resistant hypertension should be reevaluated for potential causes of secondary hypertension and considered for referral to a hypertension specialist.

CLINICS CARE POINTS

- Healthy lifestyle behaviors are a cornerstone of primary and secondary prevention of hypertension-mediated organ damage.
- Accurate blood pressure measurement is essential for the diagnosis and management of hypertension.
- Blood pressure treatment targets should be individualized based on patients' risk of cardiovascular disease and ability to safely tolerate antihypertensive therapy.
- Patients with resistant hypertension or with suspected secondary hypertension should be referred to a hypertension specialist for further evaluation.

DISCLOSURE

The authors have nothing to disclose.

SUPPLEMENTARY DATA

Supplementary data related to this article can be found online at https://doi.org/10.1016/j.cpha.2022.10.014.

REFERENCES

1. Centers for Disease Control and Prevention. High blood pressure. Available at: https://www.cdc.gov/bloodpressure/facts.htm. Accessed 20 April 2022.
2. US Preventive Services Task Force. Hypertension in adults: Screening. Available at: https://www.uspreventiveservicestaskforce.org/uspstf/recommendation/hypertension-in-adults-screening. Accessed 20 April 2022.
3. Whelton PK, Carey RM, Aronow WS, et al. 2017 ACC/AHA/AAPA/ABC/ACPM/AGS/APhA/ASH/ASPC/NMA/PCNA guideline for the prevention, detection, evaluation, and management of high blood pressure in adults: A report of the American College of Cardiology/American Heart Association task force on clinical practice guidelines. J Am Coll Cardiol 2018;71(19):e127–248. https://doi.org/10.1016/j.jacc.2017.11.006.
4. Unger T, Borghi C, Charchar F, et al. 2020 international society of hypertension global hypertension practice guidelines. Hypertension 2020;75(6):1334–57. https://doi.org/10.1161/HYPERTENSIONAHA.120.15026.
5. Pfeffer MA, Vipler B, Magee C, et al. A randomized trial of intensive versus standard blood-pressure control. N Engl J Med 2016;374(23):2290–5. https://doi.org/10.1056/NEJMc1602668.
6. Zhang W, Zhang S, Deng Y, et al. Trial of intensive blood-pressure control in older patients with hypertension. N Engl J Med 2021;385(14):1268–79. https://doi.org/10.1056/NEJMoa2111437.
7. Drawz PE, Agarwal A, Dwyer JP, et al. Concordance between blood pressure in the systolic blood pressure intervention trial and in routine clinical practice. JAMA Intern Med 2020;180(12):1655–63. https://doi.org/10.1001/jamainternmed.2020.5028.
8. Salles GF, Reboldi G, Fagard RH, et al. Prognostic effect of the nocturnal blood pressure fall in hypertensive patients: the ambulatory blood pressure collaboration in patients with hypertension (ABC-H) meta-analysis. Hypertension 2016;67(4):693–700. https://doi.org/10.1161/HYPERTENSIONAHA.115.06981.
9. Huang Q, Yang W, Asayama K, et al. Ambulatory blood pressure monitoring to diagnose and manage hypertension. Hypertension 2021;77(2):254–64. https://doi.org/10.1161/HYPERTENSIONAHA.120.14591.
10. US Blood Pressure Validated Device Listing. US blood pressure validated device listing. Available at: https://www.validatebp.org/. Accessed 20 April 2022.
11. Target BP. Patient-measured BP. Available at: https://targetbp.org/patient-measured-bp/. Accessed 20 April 2022.
12. Knauert M, Naik S, Gillespie MB, et al. Clinical consequences and economic costs of untreated obstructive sleep apnea syndrome. World J Otorhinolaryngol Head Neck Surg 2015;1(1):17–27. https://doi.org/10.1016/j.wjorl.2015.08.001.
13. Carey R, Calhoun D, Bakris G, et al. Resistant hypertension: Detection, evaluation, and management: A scientific statement from the American Heart Association. Hypertension 2018;72(5):e53–90. https://doi.org/10.1161/HYP.0000000000000084.
14. Goetsch MR, Tumarkin E, Blumenthal RS, et al. New guidance on blood pressure management in low-risk adults with stage 1 hypertension. Am Coll Cardiol 2021. Available at: https://www.acc.org/latest-in-cardiology/articles/2021/06/21/13/05/new-guidance-on-bp-management-in-low-risk-adults-with-stage-1-htn#:~:text=The%202017%20AHA%2FACC%20guidelines,%2F%3C80%20mm%20Hg. Accessed 20 April 2022.

15. Brenner BM, Cooper ME, de Zeeuw D, et al. Effects of losartan on renal and cardiovascular outcomes in patients with type 2 diabetes and nephropathy. N Engl J Med 2001;345(12):861–9. https://doi.org/10.1056/NEJMoa011161.
16. Chow CK, Atkins ER, Hillis GS, et al. Initial treatment with a single pill containing quadruple combination of quarter doses of blood pressure medicines versus standard dose monotherapy in patients with hypertension (QUARTET): A phase 3, randomised, double-blind, active-controlled trial. Lancet 2021;398(10305): 1043–52. https://doi.org/10.1016/S0140-6736(21)01922-X.
17. Pickkers P, Hughes AD, Russel FG, et al. Thiazide-induced vasodilation in humans is mediated by potassium channel activation. Hypertension 1998;32(6): 1071–6. https://doi.org/10.1161/01.hyp.32.6.1071.
18. Agarwal R, Sinha AD, Cramer AE, et al. Chlorthalidone for Hypertension in Advanced Chronic Kidney Disease. N Engl J Med 2021;385(27):2507–19. https://doi.org/10.1056/NEJMoa2110730.
19. Chen R, Suchard MA, Krumholz HM, et al. Comparative First-Line Effectiveness and Safety of ACE (Angiotensin-Converting Enzyme) Inhibitors and Angiotensin Receptor Blockers: A Multinational Cohort Study. Hypertension 2021;78(3): 591–603. https://doi.org/10.1161/HYPERTENSIONAHA.120.16667.
20. Colucci,WS, Calcium channel blockers in heart failure with reduced ejection fraction. In: UpToDate, Post TW (Ed), UpToDate, Waltham, MA. [Accessed 20 April 2022].
21. Williams B, MacDonald TM, Morant S, et al. Spironolactone versus placebo, bisoprolol, and doxazosin to determine the optimal treatment for drug-resistant hypertension (PATHWAY-2): a randomised, double-blind, crossover trial. Lancet 2015; 386(10008):2059–68. https://doi.org/10.1016/S0140-6736(15)00257-3.
22. Dudenbostel T, Calhoun DA. Resistant hypertension, obstructive sleep apnea and aldosterone. J Hum Hypertens 2012;26(5):281–7. https://doi.org/10.1038/jhh.2011.47.
23. Weiss R. Nebivolol: a novel beta-blocker with nitric oxide-induced vasodilatation. Vasc Health Risk Manag 2006;2(3):303–8. https://doi.org/10.2147/vhrm.2006.2.3.303.
24. Cheung AK, Chang TI, Cushman WC, et al. Executive summary of the KDIGO 2021 Clinical Practice Guideline for the Management of Blood Pressure in Chronic Kidney Disease. Kidney Int 2021;99(3):559–69. https://doi.org/10.1016/j.kint.2020.10.026.
25. Itoga NK, Tawfik DS, Montez-Rath ME, et al. Contributions of Systolic and Diastolic Blood Pressures to Cardiovascular Outcomes in the ALLHAT Study. J Am Coll Cardiol 2021;78(17):1671–8. https://doi.org/10.1016/j.jacc.2021.08.035.

Prescribing Across Adulthood

Kara A. Valentine, MMS, PA-C[a], Amber M. Hutchison, PharmD, BCPS, BCGP[b,*]

KEYWORDS

• Appropriate prescribing • Pharmacokinetics • Adverse drug reaction
• Medication adherence • Potentially inappropriate medications • Deprescribing
• Older adults

KEY POINTS

- The need for prescription medications is increasing because the population continues to live longer and the incidence of disease increases.
- Appropriate prescribing is a process and involves patient-centered considerations and can be accomplished by following recommended stepwise approach and applying the principles of good prescribing to the process.
- The efficacy of prescribed medications can be affected by several factors and in the older patient due to age-related physiologic changes such as pharmacokinetics, adverse drug reactions, and medication adherence.
- The identification of potentially inappropriate prescribing and deprescribing are important for the safety of the patient because there may come a point when the risk of continuing prescribed medications outweigh the benefit.

INTRODUCTION

An older adult is generally defined as being 65 years of age or older. By 2030, it is expected that 20.3% of the US population will be considered an older adult as all adults in the Baby Boomer population will be at least 65 years of age.[1] Additionally, the percentage of the population that is aged 85 years or older will double by 2036 and triple by 2049.[1] Across the life span, the goals of modern medicine include health and wellness promotion, which can assist in the reduction or prevention of illness and disease. However, when prevention cannot be done or is not achieved, other goals are the treatment and or management of disease and the relief of pain and suffering.[2] As adults age and incidence of disease increases, the use of pharmacologic agents

[a] Palm Beach Atlantic University, School of Health Professions, Physician Associate Program, 901 South Flagler Drive, West Palm Beach, FL 33401, USA; [b] Auburn University, Harrison College of Pharmacy, 1330P Walker Building, Auburn, AL 36849, USA
* Corresponding author.
E-mail address: martiam@auburn.edu

Physician Assist Clin 8 (2023) 319–328
https://doi.org/10.1016/j.cpha.2022.11.001

increases correspondingly to manage diseases, manage symptoms, or for slowing of disease progression. Pharmacologic agents can include over-the-counter (OTC) medications, prescription medications, and illicit drugs. OTC and illicit drugs are usually chosen and used at the patient's discretion, whereas prescription medications are chosen or prescribed by a medical practitioner, including physicians, physician assistants (PAs), nurse practitioners (NPs), and pharmacists.

Every practitioner must consider many factors once the decision is made to prescribe a medication. In 2002, the World Health Organization (WHO) defined rational use of medicines as, "Patients receive medications appropriate to their clinical needs, in doses that meet their own individual requirements, for an adequate period of time and at the lowest cost to them and their community."[3] If this goal is not achieved, it is considered an irrational use. Some common examples of irrational medicine use include, polypharmacy, inappropriate use of antimicrobials, not prescribing according to clinical guidelines, and inappropriate self-medicating of prescribed drugs.[3] Each of these scenarios contributes to problems in morbidity and mortality, antimicrobial resistance, and decreased trust in the health system.[3] Prescribers also play a role in the irrational use of medications. Inappropriate prescribing of medication is a concern because of the physical, mental, and financial impacts the use of prescribed medications has on the patient and the community.[3] Therefore, it is vital that prescribers implement strategies to aid in minimizing or eliminating inappropriate prescribing.

A serial retrospective cross-sectional analysis study by Jiao and colleagues compared the quality of prescribing practices of physicians and nonphysician providers, PAs and NPs, in the United States between 2006 and 2012.[4] Prescribing practices were rated based on 13 quality indicators that centered on medication use in treatment and management of chronic diseases, appropriate use of antibiotics, and appropriate prescribing in elderly patients to examine the quality of care provided.[4] The results showed all prescribers exhibited low-quality prescribing practices with no consistent difference between physicians and nonphysicians.[4] A significant limitation to this study was that it did not examine other important areas in quality prescribing such as medication monitoring and patient education.[4] This study adds to the literature that shows concern over prescribing practices in the United States.[4] This article will discuss strategies for high-quality prescribing across adulthood, including principles of appropriate prescribing, important factors to consider when prescribing in older patients, and the process of deprescribing.

Principles of Prescribing

Many national and international organizations such as the WHO, the American Academy of Family Physicians (AAFP), and the British Pharmacologic Society (BPS) have recommended systemic approaches containing core principles to guide appropriate prescribing.[5] Following these approaches will aid in reducing and eliminating inappropriate or irrational uses of medications.

The WHO's "Guide to Good Prescribing" provides guidance in a stepwise approach (**Box 1**) along with examples for rational prescribing, primarily aimed at undergraduate medical students about to start their clinical education.[6] The recommended process is intended to follow the methodology used in a good scientific experiment where there is a problem, a hypothesis, an experiment, and an outcome that undergoes verification.[6] The approach starts with the identification of the patient's problem and then the determination of specific therapeutic objectives. Once this is established, the prescriber selects an appropriate agent specifically and personally for the patient after

Box 1
Six steps in the process of rational prescribing (WHO)[6]

Step 1: Define the patient's problem.

Step 2: Specify the therapeutic objective.

Step 3: Verify whether your personal treatment plan is suitable for this patient.

Step 4: Start the treatment.

Step 5: Give information, instructions, and warnings.

Step 6: Monitor (stop) the treatment.

considering positive and negative factors and outcomes.[6] Once a suitable medication is chosen, the next step is the initiation of treatment with the prescriber providing clear patient education regarding usage information, instructions, and warnings.[6] The prescriber then determines when to monitor for results of treatment and evaluate accordingly. Once the results have been assessed, a decision on whether to continue, adjust, or discontinue treatment is made.[6]

AAFP expanded on the approach recommended by the WHO in their article titled, "Appropriate Prescribing of Medications: An Eight-Step Approach." The authors adapted the 6 steps and added 2 additional steps (**Box 2**).[5] The first additional step is to consider the cost of the medication before prescribing.[5] The last step added was to help reduce prescribing errors by using computers and other electronic tools when prescribing.[5] With the costs of health care increasing and the required use of electronic medical records for charting patient encounters, these 2 additional steps support the practice of patient-centered care and advance the goal of improving the quality of prescribing, respectively.[5] The authors also emphasize the need for ongoing self-directed learning in addition to the recommended 8-step approach to facilitate improved prescribers' quality of prescribing.[5]

The BPS published the Ten Principles of Good Prescribing to promote the safe and effective use of medications.[7] These principles align with those used in the previous stepwise approach recommendations for prescribing and include principles that factor patient-centered care and legal protection of the patient and for the prescriber.

Box 2
An 8-step approach to prescribe medications (AAFP)[5]

Step 1: Evaluate and clearly define the patient's problem.

Step 2: Specify the therapeutic objective.

Step 3: Select the appropriate drug therapy.

Step 4: Initiate therapy with appropriate details and consider nonpharmacologic therapies.

Step 5: Give information, instructions, and warnings.

Step 6: Evaluate therapy regularly.

Step 7: Consider drug cost when prescribing.

Step 8: Use computers and other tools to reduce prescribing errors.

Core principles and steps to the approach of good prescribing may be added or revised with the advancement of medicine and technology but the foundational principles remain the same. Prescribers must provide patient-centered care during the process of prescribing a medication by making decisions catered to the patients' needs and goals of treatment and consider the problem being treated, the intended outcome for treatment and what medication can help achieve intended outcome, possible outcomes for the medication chosen, the best way to educate patient on medication usage, when and how to assess outcomes from use, and whether outcomes achieved are favorable or unfavorable for intended use.

Prescribing Factors to Consider in the Older Patient

The effectiveness of a medication refers to its ability to produce a desired effect.[8] However, effectiveness does not just depend on whether the desired effect is achieved but whether it produces a patient-oriented outcome.[8] Preferred patient-oriented outcomes affecting patients' welfare include the relief of symptoms, improved function, and preservation of life.[8] Pharmacokinetics (PKs), adverse drug reactions (ADRs), and patient medication-adherence are factors that can affect the effectiveness of prescribing medications. These factors are especially of concern when prescribing for an older patient. Patient-oriented care in the older adult requires prescribers to consider medication adherence, medication cost, changes to the body due to aging and ADRs. The next sections will investigate these factors in more depth.

Pharmacokinetic Considerations

Consideration of PK changes as patients age is key when prescribing for an older adult. All medications undergo absorption, distribution, metabolism, and excretion. Each process can be affected by aging and necessitates a patient-centered approach to prescribing in older adult care.

For oral medications, absorption into the bloodstream is necessary for the medication to have its intended effect. In older adults, absorption can be affected by decreased stomach acid production or changes in intestinal transit times.[9,10]

After absorption, the medication will be distributed to its intended site of action, which depends on percent body fat, circulating proteins, and other factors. Older adults will experience a decrease in total body water, a decrease in lean muscle mass, and an increase in total body fat.[9,10] Decrease in total body water increases the concentration of a water-soluble drug, which can result in larger medication effects (both positive and negative) in older adults.[9,10] In contrast, drugs which are more lipophilic will also have an increased effect because these medications will accumulate in the increased body fat.[9,10] Changes in circulating protein is not an expected effect of aging but is affected by malnutrition. Older adults may be at risk for malnutrition due to a myriad of reasons including decreased appetite, decreased access to nutritional foods, changes in dentition, and others.[9,10] A decrease in circulating proteins will result in an increased risk of toxic effects as less drug is bound to protein and thus can exert its action on the body.[9,10]

The effects of aging on drug metabolism via the liver include changes in liver mass, hepatic blood flow, and liver enzymes.[9,10] Due to decreases in circulation, hepatic blood flow may be reduced resulting in active drug being delivered to the liver at a slower rate.[9,10] This may lead to increases in the effect of the medication due to decreased drug metabolism.[9,10] The size of the liver may also be reduced in older adults leading to a similar effect.[9,10] The activity of the liver enzymes responsible for metabolizing medications is also decreased.[9,10] All these changes may lead to an increase in the amount of time the drug is available in the body to exert its effects, which may lead to an increase in the number of ADRs related to the medications.[9,10] Unfortunately, outside the setting of chronic liver disease, the quantification of the effect of aging on hepatic metabolism is not well described.

Excretion is the last step a drug will take in the body and is accomplished through kidney and fecal elimination. Kidney elimination is a far more common pathway for elimination because drugs are often metabolized to an inert water-soluble form. Kidney function is expected to decrease somewhat as we age. Additionally, patients with various disease states may experience accelerated decreases in kidney function if their chronic diseases are not appropriately managed as they age. With decreased kidney function, exposure to medications that are eliminated by the kidneys will be increased leading to an increased risk of ADRs.[9,10] Unlike the liver, we have equations to help us estimate kidney function based on the patient's serum creatinine. The most used currently are the Cockcroft-Gault formula for estimating creatinine clearance and CKD-EPI 2021 SCr equation for estimating the glomerular filtration rate. Using these equations, all medications should be regularly evaluated for dosing adjustments related to kidney function.[9,10]

Physical Changes Related to the Older Adult

Throughout the aging process, changes take place in the body, which may directly or indirectly affect the use of medications in older adults. Changes in manual dexterity due to various reasons including arthritis can influence the use of medications via difficulties in medication administration, particularly dosage forms such as eye drops, injectable products, or other dosage forms requiring coordination.[9] Visual changes in the older adult may also affect medication use through difficulties in identifying medications.[9] Patients may require alternative methods to identify and manage their medications. Finally, hearing loss may affect the ability to receive medication education and may require adjustment on behalf of the health-care provider to ensure a conducive environment for delivery.[9]

Increased Risk for Adverse Drug Reactions

The WHO defines an ADR as "a response to a drug that is noxious and unintended and occurs at doses normally used in man for the prophylaxis, diagnosis or therapy of disease, or for modification of physiological function."[11] ADRs can affect a patient's ability to continue with treatment and, particularly in the older patient, may also cause additional medical problems. Some common clinical presentations of ADRs in the older patient include falls, kidney failure, orthostatic hypotension, delirium, and bleeding (particularly gastrointestinal and intracranial).[12] An adverse drug event (ADE) occurs when a person is harmed due to the use of a medication.[13] The Centers for Disease Control reports that older adults visit the emergency department due to an ADE approximately 450,000 times annually at a rate, which is more than twice that of younger patients.[13]

As estimates show that almost half of ADEs are avoidable, and prescribers have a responsibility to evaluate for possible ADEs before prescribing a medication to an older patient.[14] ADE risk assessments can be done with prospective, concurrent, and retrospective surveillance systems.[15] Prospective surveillance involves the monitoring of patients with high risk for ADRs and monitoring patients taking medications with an increased potential for causing ADRs before initiating treatment with a new medication.[15] Risk factors for ADEs can be categorized as patient-specific, drug-specific, and clinician-specific.[14] Polypharmacy (defined in a later section) is an example of an ADE that can fall into any of these 3 risk categories and is possibly the strongest risk factor for ADEs in older adults.[15] Patient-specific risk factors include extremes of ages, history of allergy or previous ADR, pharmacodynamic or PK changes, the presence of concurrent disease states, and severity of illness.[15] Drug-specific risk factors are based on classes of medications known to have an increased risk for causing ADRs. These include anticoagulants, antimicrobials, antidiabetic agents, cardiac agents, and central nervous system agents.[15] More than 50% of Medicare patients visit the emergency department due to ADEs with antidiabetic agents, oral anticoagulants, antiplatelet agents, and opioid pain medications combined.[14] Concurrent surveillance involves the recognition of an ADR close to when it manifests.[15] Retrospective surveillance involves the evaluation of medical records for the occurrence of an ADR; however, this method has some disadvantages, namely delayed identification of and reaction to ADRs.[15]

To help reduce and prevent ADEs from occurring, safety measures for prescribing medications should occur during the ordering, transcribing, dispensing, and administrating phases.[14] Prescribers should have a heightened index of suspicion for possible ADRs in patients that develop new symptoms after the start of a new medication or after a dosage change, especially in the case of older patients.[12] In the older patient, ADRs contribute significantly to these patients' morbidity and mortality, therefore, careful monitoring and regular review of all pharmacologic agents is essential.[12]

Medication Nonadherence

Medication adherence refers to the extent to which a patients' behavior in taking a prescribed medication corresponds with the recommendations of the prescriber.[16] It has been estimated nonadherence causes approximately 125,000 preventable deaths annually.[17] As this causes significant mortality, it is key for prescribers to assess adherence rather than assuming patients are taking medications as instructed. When addressing the issue of nonadherence, prescribers should be aware that medication adherence is a multifaceted and multidimensional issue and should be cognizant of whether it is intentional or unintentional.[16] Unfortunately, prescribers often ignore this issue or think it is a personal problem of the patient rather than acknowledging it, which may additionally be a prescriber or health system problem.[18] Currently, the focus on improving this issue relies on addressing barriers to adherence that can be patient-related, treatment-related, and prescriber-related.[18]

Some patient-related barriers to medication adherence include lack of motivation, cultural differences, alternate belief systems, feelings of depression and/or denial, and low educational level.[18] A few treatment-related barriers include cost, time, inconvenience, side effects or the fear thereof, and complexity of treatment.[18] A prescriber-related barrier is poor practitioner–patient relationship.[18] The older patient is more susceptible to having additional factors contributing to nonadherence like changes or decline in cognition, loss of manual dexterity, and lack of social support.[19]

Polypharmacy and Deprescribing

Polypharmacy is generally defined as the use of multiple medications with quantitative definitions including 2 or greater to greater than 11 medications as benchmarks.[20] Reports show that most older adults use at least one prescription medication daily and 35.8% of community-dwelling older adults use 5 or more prescription medications daily.[21] Polypharmacy can lead to increased health-care costs, increased risk of ADEs, and other serious consequences.[22] Although some disease states require multiple medications to manage the patient's condition, many older adults may be prescribed inappropriate medications. Managing polypharmacy requires identifying potentially inappropriate medications (PIMs) followed by appropriate deprescribing.

Table 1
Currently published deprescribing and PIMs tools

Criteria	Brief Description	Published Literature
Beers criteria	List of PIMs and other clinical considerations	The 2019 American Geriatrics Society Beers Criteria® Update Expert Panel. American Geriatrics Society 2019 updated AGS Beers Criteria® for potentially inappropriate medication use in older adults. J Am Geriar Soc 2019;67(4):674–694
STOPP tool	Identifies PIMs arranged by organ system	Hamilton HJ, Gallagher PF, O'Mahony D. Inappropriate prescribing and adverse drug events in older people. BMC Geriatr 2009;9:5
EU-(7) PIM list	A list of PIMs in Europe	Renom-Guiteras A, Meyer G, Thurmann. The EU(7)-PIM list: a list of potentially inappropriate medications for older people consented by experts from seven European countries. Eur J Clin Pharmacol 2015;71(7):861–75
Garfinkel Good Palliative-Geriatric Practice (GPGP) method	An implicit method for deprescribing	Bilek AJ, Levy Y, Kab H, et al. Teaching physicians the GPGP method promotes deprescribing in both inpatient and outpatient settings. Ther Adv Drug Saf 2019;10:1–16
McLeod criteria	A list of inappropriate prescribing practices developed as a Canadian consensus guideline	McLeod PJ, Huang AR, Tamblyn RM, et al. Defining inappropriate practices in prescribing for elderly people: a national consensus panel. CMAJ 1997;156(3):385–91
Medication inappropriateness index	Ten scored questions to determine if a medication is inappropriate. Mostly used in research	Hanlon JT, Schmader KE, Samsa GP, et al. A method for assessing drug therapy appropriateness. J Clin Epidemiol 1992;45(10):1045–51
Fit for the aged criteria (FORTA)	Drug classification system giving medications in main indication groups a score for necessity of medication	Kuhn-Thiel AM, Wei C, Wehline M, et al. Consensus validation of the FORTA List: a clinical tool for increasing the appropriateness of pharmacotherapy in the elderly. Drugs Aging 2014;31(2):131–40

Box 3
The deprescribing protocol[25]

1. Compile a complete and current medication list along with reasons for each medication.
2. Evaluate the risk of ADEs.
3. Assess each drug for the potential to be discontinued.
4. Prioritize drugs for discontinuation.
5. Implement and monitor drug discontinuation regimen.

PIMs are medications that may not be beneficial in older adults.[23] The American Geriatrics Society Beers Criteria is perhaps the most widely known and recognized set of criteria for PIMs in older adults.[23] These criteria can be applied to patients aged older than 65 years in both ambulatory and institutional settings but they do not apply to palliative and hospice care patients.[23] Medications are included in the Beers Criteria if published literature shows a poor risk-to-benefit ratio in older adults.[23] The criteria also indicate the quality of evidence and the strength of the recommendation, which may be helpful in considering deprescribing.[23] The tables in the Beers Criteria are the major focus of the reference and provide detailed information regarding PIMs and other general medication considerations for older adults. The evidence is graded based on quality of evidence and the strength of the recommendation.[23] When using the Beers Criteria, it is important to remember that PIMs may be appropriate in some situations.[23,24] It is most helpful to use the Beers Criteria to identify potentially problematic medications and offer appropriate alternatives as clinically appropriate for the patient.[23,24]

The identification of PIMs should follow with a careful clinical evaluation of the use of the medication and then proceed with deprescribing as appropriate.[23] Deprescribing is defined as "the systematic process of identifying and discontinuing drugs in instances in which existing or potential harms outweigh existing or potential benefits within the context of an individual patient's care goals, current level of functioning, life expectancy, values, and preferences."[25] There are several tools available for deprescribing considerations (**Table 1**). It is important to note that deprescribing criteria and PIMs lists do not condone preventing the appropriate management of patients and their disease burden but instead focus on appropriate and timely usage of medications. Deprescribing should always be considered and is especially important for older adults on multiple medications. A 5-step process for deprescribing has been proposed by Scott and colleagues and can be found in **Box 3**.

Any deprescribing should be accompanied by consultation with the patient and the patient's goals of therapy along with counseling regarding the medication changes.[23,25] Additionally, it may be prudent to discuss medication destruction with the patient as necessary, especially because it relates to controlled substances.

SUMMARY

Prescribing across the life span should be done methodically using a patient-centered approach. This is especially true for older adults who may experience disproportionate difficulties in their medication management. When prescribing medications to older adults, PK and physiologic changes should be accounted for all current medications and future medications. There are several tools available for the identification of PIMs along with tools for deprescribing as appropriate.

CLINICS CARE POINTS

- Clinicians should consider prescribing medications as a process and ensure that each step is completed before a patient-centered team-based decision is made.
- The implementation of recommended prescribing strategies can be used to minimize or eliminate inappropriate prescribing, which can be harmful to the patient as well as the community.
- Prescribers must continuously monitor whether prescribed medications are effective and achieve preferred patient-oriented outcomes, as well as consider factors that can affect effectiveness, including pharmacokinetics, adverse drug reactions, and patient medication-adherence.
- Clinicians should continuously evaluate for PIMs and initiate deprescribing when appropriate in the efforts to reduce inappropriate polypharmacy, especially in the elderly.

DISCLOSURE

The authors declared no potential conflicts of interests to the research, authorship, and/or publication of this article.

REFERENCES

1. Ortman JM, Velkoff Va, Hogan H. An aging nation: the older population in the United States 2014. Available at: https://www.census.gov/library/publications/2014/demo/p25-1140.html. Accessed May 5, 2022.
2. Callahan D. Managed care and the goals of medicine. J Am Geriatr Soc 1998;46(3):385–8.
3. World Health Organization. Promoting rational use of medicines: core components. 2002. Available at: https://apps.who.int/iris/bitstream/handle/10665/67438/WHO_EDM_2002.3.pdf. Accessed May 5, 2022.
4. Jiao W, Murimi IB, Stafford RS, et al. Quality of prescribing by physicians, nurse practitioners, and physician assistants in the United States. Pharmacotherapy 2018;38(4):417–27.
5. Pollock M, Bazaldua OV, Dobbie AE. Appropriate prescribing of medications: an eight-step approach. Am Fam Physician 2007;75(2):231–6.
6. De Vries TP, Henning RH, Hogerzeil HV, et al. Guide to good prescribing: a practical manual. 1994. Available at: https://apps.who.int/iris/bitstream/handle/10665/59001/WHO_DAP_94.11.pdf. Accessed May 2, 2022.
7. British Pharmacological Society. Ten principles of good prescribing. 2022. Available at: https://www.bps.ac.uk/education-engagement/teaching-pharmacology/ten-principles-of-good-prescribing. Accessed May 2, 2022.
8. Lynch SS. Drug efficacy and safety. 2019. Available at: https://www.merckmanuals.com/professional/clinical-pharmacology/concepts-in-pharmacotherapy/drug-efficacy-and-safety#v8423102. Accessed May 2, 2022.
9. Hutchison LC. Biomedical principles of aging. In: Hutchison LC, Sleeper RB, editors. Fundamentals of geriatric pharmacotherapy: an evidence-based approach. 2nd edition. Bethesda: ASHP; 2015. p. 57–76.
10. Wooten JM. Pharmacotherapy considerations in elderly adults. South Med J 2012;105(8):437–45.
11. Report of a WHO Meeting. International drug monitoring: the role of national centres. World Health Organ Tech Rep Ser 1972;498:1–25.

12. Lavan QH, Gallagher P. Predicting risk of adverse drug reactions in older adults. Ther Adv Drug Saf 2016;7(1):11–22.
13. Centers for Disease Control. Adverse drug events in adults. 2017. Available at: https://www.cdc.gov/medicationsafety/adult_adversedrugevents.html. Accessed May 4, 2022.
14. Agency for Healthcare Research and Quality. Medication errors and adverse drug events. Available at: https://psnet.ahrq.gov/primer/medication-errors-and-adverse-drug-events. Accessed May 4, 2022.
15. Murdaugh LB. Adverse drug reaction reporting. In: Competence assessment tools. 5th edition. Bethesda: ASHP; 2015. p. 545–56.
16. Hugtenburg JG, Timmers L, Elders PJ, et al. Definitions, variants, and causes of nonadherence with medication: a challenge for tailored interventions. Patient Prefer Adherence 2013;7:675–82.
17. Boylan L. The cost of medication non-adherence. 2017. Available at: https://www.nacds.org/news/the-cost-of-medication-non-adherence/. Accessed May 4, 2022.
18. Kleinsinger F. The unmet challenge of medication nonadherence. Perm J 2018;22:18–033.
19. Steinman MA, Holmes HM. Principles of prescribing & adherence. In: Walter LC, Chang A, Chen P, et al, editors. Current diagnosis & treatment geriatrics. 3rd ed. McGraw Hill; 2021. Available at: https://accessmedicine.mhmedical.com/content.aspx?bookid=2984&sectionid=250007024. Accessed March 07, 2022.
20. Masnoon N, Shakib S, Kalish-Ellett L, et al. What is polypharmacy: a systematic review of definitions. Geriatrics 2017;17:230–40.
21. Qato DM, Wilder J, Schumm LP, et al. Changes in prescription and over-the-counter medication and dietary supplement use among older adults in the United States, 2005 vs. 2011. JAMA Intern Med 2016;176(4):473–82.
22. Maher RL, Hanlon JT, Hajjar ER. Clinical consequences of polypharmacy in elderly. Expert Opin Drug Saf 2014;13(1):57–65.
23. The 2019 American Geriatrics Society Beers Criteria® Update Expert Panel. American Geriatrics Society 2019 updated AGS Beers Criteria® for potentially inappropriate medication use in older adults. J Am Geriar Soc 2019;67(4):674–94.
24. Steinman MA. Using wisely: a reminder on the proper use of the American Geriatrics Society Beers Criteria. J Am Geriatr Soc 2019;67(4):644–6.
25. Scott IA, Hilmer SN, Reeve E, et al. Reducing inappropriate polypharmacy: the process of deprescribing. JAMA Intern Med 2015;175(5):827–34.

Pain Management in the Opioid Crisis

Valerie Prince, PharmD, BCPS[a,b,*]

KEYWORDS

• Opioids • Pain • Tapering • Crisis • CDC

KEY POINTS

- The opioid crisis presents challenges for managing patients with pain.
- The 2016 Centers for Disease Control (CDC) Opioid Prescribing Guidelines were frequently applied incorrectly.
- New CDC Opioid Prescribing Guidelines are expected in 2022.
- Rapid opioid tapers or sudden discontinuation poses many dangers for patients.
- Adjunctive agents are available and useful for opioid-sparing effects.

INTRODUCTION

The opioid epidemic has been a growing threat to lives in our society for much longer than the COVID pandemic. The number of drug overdose deaths has quadrupled since 1999.[1] From 2018 to 2019, opioid-involved death rates increased by over 6% and synthetic opioid-involved death rates (excluding methadone) increased by over 15% which are staggering increases in patient harm.[2] Origins of this epidemic are complex. One major contributing factor was the false reassurance to the medical community by pharmaceutical companies that patients being treated for pain would not become "addicted" to opioids. Opioid prescribing increased in the late 1900s due in part to this false sense of security. Increased use of prescription opioids led to misuse of both prescription and illicit opioids. Soon, it became clear that opioid analgesics were correlated with the development of substance use disorders. In 2017, the US Department of Health and Human Services (HHS) declared that the opioid crisis was a public health emergency. In addition to the devastating consequences of the opioid epidemic in adults, the crisis resulted in a rising incidence of newborns experiencing withdrawal syndrome due to opioid use and misuse during pregnancy.[3] The opioid epidemic greatly complicates care for patients with pain.

[a] Samford University McWhorter School of Pharmacy, Samford University, 800 Lakeshore Drive, Birmingham, AL 35229, USA; [b] St Vincent's East Family Medicine Residency Program, Christ Health Center, 110 Lakeside Drive, Odenville, AL 35120, USA
* Corresponding author. Samford University, 800 Lakeshore Drive, Birmingham, AL 35229.
E-mail address: vtprince@samford.edu

Physician Assist Clin 8 (2023) 329–338
https://doi.org/10.1016/j.cpha.2022.10.010

Both appropriate and inappropriate prescribing of opioids contribute to the current crisis. Appropriate prescribing for patients with pain can unintentionally result in the development of substance use disorders or overdose. Overprescribing opioids for pain also results in more opioids available for diversion and misuse. Responsible opioid use is a challenge for healthcare providers in the face of patients with chronic pain especially.

In addition to overdose and substance use disorders, there are other reasons why searching for alternative forms of pain management is important. As early as 1870, medical literature described a paradoxical phenomenon of increased sensitivity to pain in the presence of opioids. This phenomenon, then described as "morphia", is now termed opioid-induced hyperalgesia. Opioid-induced hyperalgesia is a major complicating factor in the treatment of pain with opioids. Some experts have speculated that overtreatment with opioids might have contributed to the rise in chronic pain in the United States. Most of the world's prescription opioids are consumed by Americans, whereas most developed countries have a lower pain prevalence than the United States. It is incumbent on the healthcare community to find the line between facilitating opioid misuse and appropriately treating patients with pain. In our efforts to do so, we have often stigmatized patients as "addicts" or placed limitations on patients' ability to access the opioids they need.[4]

Nonopioid Therapeutic Options

Because of drawbacks in opioid therapy, an important area of inquiry in the field of pain management is the use of adjunctive agents. These agents were often not originally approved to manage pain but there is evidence that select adjuvants are effective as analgesics in certain disease states. Nonopioid adjunctive analgesics can play an important role in both efficacy and safety. Adjunctive analgesics can enhance the effect of analgesia when a patient's response to opioid treatment decreases and they can help minimize unwanted adverse effects. Some of these agents can have an opioid dose-sparing effect when used as part of a multimodal approach to address pain. In some circumstances, alternative agents can be used rather than in addition to opioids. Providers may not have an accurate understanding of the efficacy, harms, and role in pain therapy these medications can provide.

Non-steroidal Anti-inflammatory Drugs

One of the medication classes with a great deal of utility in pain management is non-steroidal anti-inflammatory drugs (NSAIDs). Providers may be hesitant to use NSAIDs due to their perceived toxicity relative to opioids. In actuality, when accounting for all adverse events, a Cochrane Collaborative meta-analysis of 350 randomized trials showed that opioids had double the rate of adverse events of NSAIDs.[5] They are very effective analgesics when used in a variety of clinical scenarios. The American Academy of Otolaryngology–Head and Neck Surgery Clinical Practice Guideline, "Opioid Prescribing for Analgesia After Common Otolaryngology Operations," recommends multimodal nonopioid analgesics such as NSAIDs as first-line therapy.[6] Use of NSAIDs and other adjuvants has been studied in critical care environments as well. A 2020 systemic review of multiple adjuvants in critical care environments found that the use of any adjuvant studied, NSAIDs in addition to an opioid led to reductions in both patient-reported pain scores and opioid consumption at 24 hours.[7] The American Pain Society and the American Society of Anesthesiologists advocate the use of a multimodal pain management strategy.[8] Nonopioid medications are used in enhanced recovery after surgery (ERAS) protocols to provide effective analgesia while sparing opioid administration. ERAS emphasizes avoidance of adverse medication reactions such as nausea, pruritis, and sedation during recovery.[9] Reducing opioid side effects could potentially positively impact patients' length of stay. Perioperative care teams are well-positioned to implement new clinical strategies that balance appropriate pain management and opioid diversion prevention.[10]

Duloxetine and Venlafaxine

Duloxetine and venlafaxine are serotonin-norepinephrine reuptake inhibitors often used for psychiatric conditions and pain. Both agents can be useful adjuvants or alternatives to opioids and/or NSAIDs depending on the type of pain. Duloxetine is a first-line choice for the treatment of neuropathic pain syndromes like diabetic neuropathy. Additional indications for duloxetine include low back and non-radicular neck pain, fibromyalgia, and osteoarthritis of the knee when non-pharmacological approaches plus NSAIDs have failed to control symptoms. Nausea often occurs with duloxetine necessitating starting with a low dose and titrating up as tolerated. Venlafaxine has a different adverse effect profile and may contribute to hypertension at higher doses. Venlafaxine also indicates use in diabetic neuropathic pain.[11] See **Table 1** for dosing information on select adjuvants.

Gabapentin and Pregabalin

Gabapentin and Pregabalin are anticonvulants which are first-line choices in the management of neuropathic pain.[12] A major drawback to the use of both of these drugs is a well-documented potential for abuse. Although these drugs are not opioids, their abuse is often related to opioid abuse. In addition to getting high, other main reasons people abuse these drugs are to ease opioid withdrawal symptoms and increase the effects of methadone.[13] Pregabalin has been classified as a controlled substance by the Drug Enforcement Administration which indicates significant evidence for abuse potential and physiologic dependence.[14] Both drugs should be tapered off over a minimum period of 1 week to prevent a withdrawal syndrome. In addition to abuse liability, both drugs share adverse effects of weight gain edema, dizziness, and somnolence.

Tricyclic Antidepressants

Tricyclic antidepressants (TCAs) as a drug class are considered first-line options for neuropathic pain.[12] This class of drugs has many known adverse effects that may limit their use. TCAs are not recommended for use in patients with cardiovascular disease and should only be used with caution in the elderly due to anticholinergic effects.

Table 1
Opioid dosing for select oral opioids

Opioid	Initial Dose (Opioid-Naïve)	Max Total Daily Dose (Outpatient Setting)
Morphine (IR)[38]	10 mg q4h	As tolerated
Codeine/Acetaminophen[39]	30/300 mg q4h	360/1800 mg/d
Hydrocodone/Acetaminophen[40]	5/325 mg q6h	Product specific: max acetaminophen dose is 4000 mg/d
Oxycodone (IR)[41]	5 mg q6h	30 mg/d
Hydromorphone[42]	1 mg q6h	12 mg/d

Abbreviation: IR, immediate release.

Skeletal Muscle Relaxants

One class of medications being used as adjuvants in ERAS protocols are skeletal muscle relaxants (SMRs). Skeletal muscle relaxants are used in a variety of pain states such as fibromyalgia, low back pain, and neuropathic pain.[15] The exact mechanism of action is not fully elucidated for many SMRs such as cyclobenzaprine, metaxalone, and methocarbamol.[16]

Atypical Antipsychotics

Atypical antipsychotics have been explored as adjunctive pain agents. A review published in 2021 revealed that both olanzapine and quetiapine were able to decrease pain scores on the numeric rating scale, indicating a reduction in pain experienced. Craving behavior was also reduced. Quetiapine was shown to improve depression scores and quality-of-life indicators.[17]

Opioid Pharmacology

Opioids are derived from the poppy plant (which is also the source of heroin) and are designed to provide relief from pain. Many prescribers are wary of prescribing opioids for good reason. Opioids for both acute and chronic pain have been linked to the development of misuse, abuse, adverse drug effects, and opioid use disorder in patients. Other adverse effects of opioids can include respiratory depression, constipation, immunosuppression, hyperalgesia, and other gastrointestinal disturbances. Opioids produce their pharmacologic actions by acting on the mu, delta, and kappa receptors located on neuronal cell membrane receptors that lead to supraspinal analgesia and potential opioid adverse effects. Chronic use of opioids is associated with increased tolerance, and decreasing analgesic effects requiring an increase in dosing.[18] See **Table 2** for dosing recommendations for select oral opioids.

2016 Centers for Disease Control Opioids for Chronic Pain Guidelines

In response to the opioid crisis, the CDC developed a set of opioid prescribing guidelines in 2016. In the decade preceding the guidelines, deaths from prescription pain medication had increased markedly whereas other leading causes of death such as heart disease and cancer had decreased.[19] From 2007 to 2013, opioid prescribing increased overall with family medicine, general medicine, and internal medicine having greater increases than other specialties.[20] Additionally at the time of the review for the 2016 guidelines no evidence showed a long-term benefit of opioids in pain and function versus no opioids for chronic pain with outcomes examined at least 1 year later.[21,22] All these factors and others led to the development of the CDC Guidelines for Prescribing Opioids for Chronic Pain.[23] See **Box 1** for selected guidelines. These guidelines were intended to facilitate safer prescribing for primary care providers in the treatment of adult patients with chronic pain outside of active cancer treatment, palliative care, and end-of-life care. Uptake and misapplication of these guidelines

Table 2
Dosing for select adjuvants for treating neuropathic pain

Medication	Initial Dose	Titration	Max Total Daily Dose
Venlafaxine[11]	37.5 mg/d	Weekly	225 mg/d
Duloxetine[43]	30 mg/d	Weekly	60 mg/d
Gabapentin[44]	100 mg/d	1–2 wk	3.6 gm/d divided
Pregabalin[45]	75 mg BID	Weekly	600 mg/d divided

Box 1
Select recommendations from CDC guidelines on opioid prescribing for chronic pain, 2016

- Nonpharmacologic therapy and nonopioid pharmacologic therapy are preferred for chronic pain. Clinicians should consider opioid therapy only if the expected benefits for both pain and function are anticipated to outweigh risks to the patient. If opioids are used, they should be combined with nonpharmacologic therapy and nonopioid pharmacologic therapy, as appropriate.
- Clinicians should evaluate benefits and harms with patients within 1 to 4 weeks of starting opioid therapy for chronic pain or dose escalation. Clinicians should evaluate the benefits and harms of continued therapy with patients every 3 months or more frequently. If the benefits do not outweigh the harms of continued opioid therapy, clinicians should optimize other therapies and work with patients to taper opioids to lower dosages or to taper and discontinue opioids.
- Clinicians should avoid prescribing opioid pain medication and benzodiazepines concurrently whenever possible.
- Clinicians should offer or arrange evidence-based treatment (usually medication-assisted treatment with buprenorphine or methadone in combination with behavioral therapies) for patients with opioid-use disorder.
- Before starting and periodically during the continuation of opioid therapy, clinicians should evaluate risk factors for opioid-related harms. Clinicians should incorporate into the management plan strategies to mitigate risk, including considering offering naloxone when factors that increase the risk for opioid overdose, such as the history of overdose, history of a substance use disorder, higher opioid dosages (≥50 MME/d), or concurrent benzodiazepine use, are present.

were rapid. Inappropriate policies and practices developed that went far beyond the actual recommendations or were not concordant with the guidelines. The CDC guidelines clearly stated individual judgment should be used based on a cautious assessment of benefits vs. risks regarding many aspects of opioid prescribing. Two of those aspects are dosage and duration thresholds. The guidelines included information on "morphine milligram equivalents (MME)" An MME is the amount of morphine to which an opioid dose is equal when prescribed. The guidelines suggested a cautious assessment of benefits vs. risks when considering increasing dosage to ≥50 MME/day, and carefully justifying a decision to titrate dosage to ≥90 MME/day. (See resources for a link to an online MME/day calculator.) Unfortunately, dosage and duration thresholds were misinterpreted as hard limits resulting in abrupt tapering of drugs, patients receiving inadequate treatment, and patient dismissal from medical practices. These dosages and duration thresholds were also incorrectly applied to populations such as patients with opioid use disorders (OUD), cancer, sickle cell, and those undergoing surgical procedures.[24]

Many other problems resulted from guideline misapplication including lack of availability and coverage for comprehensive multimodal pain management. In a multimodal approach, adjuvant agents may be used in addition to, rather than instead of, an opioid. Misapplication led to barriers to access evidence-based OUD treatment and underutilization of naloxone. One of the most dangerous challenges arising from misinterpretation of the 2016 CDC Opioid Prescribing Guidelines is the abrupt cessation of opioids in patients who have developed the expected physical dependency on opioids. Physical dependency occurs when the body becomes accustomed to the presence of a drug and the patient experiences a withdrawal syndrome when the drug is stopped. This is a recognized effect for many classes of medications such as beta-blockers, steroids, and opioids. Physical dependency may be one component of an OUD but the presence of it alone in the absence of other diagnostic criteria does not indicate an OUD.[25] Policies to restrict daily doses have been enacted in several states. Also, private insurers have limited coverage to control and limit doses.[26] In response to these misapplications as well as new literature available to inform guidelines, the CDC developed an updated guideline that is currently posted on the Federal Register to solicit comments from anyone (healthcare providers, public, and so forth) who would like to provide input. The new guidelines are expected to be finalized by the end of 2022.[27]

Opioid Tapering

One dangerous practice attributed to the misapplication of the CDC guidelines is rapid tapering or abruptly discontinuing opioids. An expert panel was convened to explore literature related to the misapplication of the CDC guidelines. The panel was unanimous that abrupt cessation of opioids (and sedatives) is not the intent of the CDC guidelines and is not safe for the patient. These experts commented that it is unacceptable practice to abruptly dismiss physically-dependent patients from care. They stipulated that an adequate plan for pain or OUD treatment is a necessary follow-up except in unusual circumstances, such as diversion. Some prescribers may be unaware of the detailed discussion provided by the CDC guidelines regarding the need for gentle and often slow tapers. The CDC Opioid Prescribing Guidelines Recommendation #7 supports a decision based on an individualized evaluation of harm versus benefit. This recommendation does not mandate taper to any target. The panel affirmed that providers should offer a gentle taper with corresponding attention to ensuring alternative pain treatments or OUD treatment if needed is available. If the provider is unwilling or unable to attend to these issues, they have an obligation to refer the patient to a provider willing to provide these services.[28,29]

In recognition of this dangerous misapplication of CDC Opioid Prescribing Guidelines, the US Department of HHS published guidelines on opioid tapering in 2019. These guidelines included information on the risks associated with rapid opioid dose reductions. In addition to somatic withdrawal symptoms, rapid tapers are associated with significant psychological distress. These guidelines also warned of the risk of patients transitioning to illicit opioids.[30] It is an emotional ordeal for many patients to experience the tapering process, and both the HHS and CDC guidelines advise clinicians to monitor patients carefully during tapering and to provide psychosocial support.[31,32] One of the many dangers of rapid tapers is opioid overdose. Patients who do not understand the concept of tolerance during a taper may try to resume original doses or take illicit substances to replace the opioid being tapered. A study published in Journal of the American Medical Association (JAMA) in 2021 revealed that tapering was significantly associated with absolute differences in rates of overdose or mental health crisis compared with not tapering.[33]

Impact of Opioid Crisis on Patients with Chronic Pain

Patients who are prescribed chronic opioid therapy are frequently disadvantaged and looked down on in our healthcare system. Consequently, these patients suffer negative consequences, such as delayed or missed diagnosis, bias in treatment, barriers in care, and inadequate care. A lack of understanding of the difference between an OUD and physical dependence on an opioid has contributed to the stigma. Moreover, literature has reported unfavorable effectiveness and functional improvement outcomes for patients who are treated long-term with opioids. Many negative outcomes in addition to abuse have been documented in patients who are treated long-term with opioids.[22,34–37] Opioid therapy can be minimized by using alternative agents and/or a multimodal approach to managing pain. In a multimodal approach, drugs from different classes are included in the regimen to minimize or eliminate opioid use. Non-pharmacological interventions can also be an important component of a multimodal regimen.

SUMMARY

Prescribing opioids appropriately to the correct patients is difficult in today's health-care environment. Multiple insurance providers, state boards, and national pharmacy chains have enacted opioid limits that result in barriers to chronic pain patients and their providers. The National Institutes of Drug Abuse (NIDA) published safe prescribing practices to help practitioners safely provide opioids. The NIDA recognizes that opioids may be appropriate for some patients with severe pain. If opioids are necessary for a patient, there are several concepts to remember to use these medications as safely as possible.

- Prescribe the lowest effective dose to decrease the chances of an overdose, death, or the development of an OUD (**Table 2**).
- Avoid if possible co-prescribing opioids and benzodiazepines or SMRs.
- Limit the duration of opioid therapy to no longer than absolutely necessary.

Literature shows us that about half of the patients who take opioids for more than 30 days in the first year will continue to take them for at least 3 years. Patients with central pain syndromes, such as fibromyalgia and tension headaches, respond better to antidepressants and anticonvulsants than to opioids. Carefully re-evaluate the risk versus benefit of continued opioid therapy after a non-fatal overdose. Use CDC Opioid Prescribing Guidelines as evidence-based suggestions for the safer use of these drugs.

CLINICS CARE POINTS

- Rapid opioid tapers are associated with somatic withdrawal symptoms, psychological distress, transition to illicit opioids and overdose deaths.
- The American Pain Society and the American Society of Anesthesiologists advocate use of a multimodal pain managment strategy.
- Opioids have double the rate of adverse events compared to NSAIDs.

DISCLOSURE

The author (V. Prince) has no commercial or financial conflicts of interest or any funding sources to disclose.

REFERENCES

1. Centers for Disease Control and Prevention. Wide-ranging online data for epidemiologic research (WONDER). Atlanta, GA: CDC, National Center for Health Statistics; 2020. Available at: http://wonder.cdc.gov. Accessed May 27, 2022.
2. Mattson CL, Tanz LJ, Quinn K, et al. Trends and geographic patterns in drug and synthetic opioid overdose deaths — United States, 2013–2019. MMWR Morb Mortal Wkly Rep 2021;70:202–7.

3. U.S. Department of Health and Human Services. What is the U.S. opioid epidemic?. Available at: https://www.hhs.gov/opioids/about-the-epidemic/index.html. Accessed May 27, 2022.
4. National Institute on Drug Abuse. Responsibly and sensitively addressing chronic pain amid an opioid crisis. NIDA; 2016. Available at: https://archives.drugabuse.gov/about-nida/noras-blog/2016/09/responsibly-sensitively-addressing-chronic-pain-amid-opioid-crisis. Accessed May 31, 2022.
5. Moore RA, Derry S, Aldington D, et al. Adverse events associated with single dose oral analgesics for acute postoperative pain in adults: an overview of Cochrane reviews. Cochrane Database Syst Rev 2015;10:CD011407.
6. Anne S, Mims JW, Tunkel DE, et al. Clinical practice guideline: opioid prescribing for analgesia after common otolaryngology operations executive summary. Otolaryngol Head Neck Surg 2021;164(4):687–703.
7. Wheeler KE, Grilli R, Centofanti JE, et al. Adjuvant analgesic use in the critically ill: A systematic review and meta-analysis. Crit Care Explor 2020;2(7):e0157. Published 2020 Jul 6.
8. Chou R, Gordon DB, de Leon-Casasola OA, et al. Management of postoperative pain: a clinical practice guideline from the American Pain Society, the American Society of Regional Anesthesia and Pain Medicine, and the American Society of Anesthesiologists' Committee on Regional Anesthesia, Executive Committee, and Administrative Council. J Pain 2016;17(2):131–57.
9. Bhatia A, Buvanendran A. Anesthesia and postoperative pain control-multimodal anesthesia protocol. J Spine Surg 2019;5(Suppl 2):S160–5.
10. Hah JM, Bateman BT, Ratliff J, et al. Chronic opioid use after surgery: implications for perioperative management in the face of the opioid epidemic. Anesth Analg 2017;125(5):1733–40.
11. Venlafaxine. Lexi-drugs. Hudson, OH: Lexicomp; 2022. Available at: http://online.lexi.com/. Accessed May 27, 2022.
12. Fornasari D. Pharmacotherapy for neuropathic pain: a review. Pain Ther 2017;6(Suppl 1):25–33.
13. Quintero G. Review about gabapentin misuse, interactions, contraindications and side effects. J Exp Pharmacol 2017;9:13–21.
14. United States Drug Enforcement Administration. Drug Scheduling. Available from. https://www.dea.gov/drug-information/drug-scheduling. Accessed May 30, 2022.
15. Chou R, Peterson K, Helfand M. Comparative efficacy and safety of skeletal muscle relaxants for spasticity and musculoskeletal conditions: a systematic review. J Pain Symptom Manage 2004;28(2):140–75.
16. See S, Ginzburg R. Skeletal Muscle Relaxants. Pharmacotherapy 2008;28(2):207–13.
17. Coronado B, Dunn J, Veronin MA, et al. Efficacy and safety considerations with second-generation antipsychotics as adjunctive analgesics: a review of literature. J Pharm Technol 2021;37(4):202–8.
18. Dhaliwal A, Gupta M. Physiology, opioid receptor. [Updated 2021 Jul 26]. In: StatPearls [internet]. Treasure Island (FL): StatPearls Publishing; 2022. Available from: https://www.ncbi.nlm.nih.gov/books/NBK546642/. Accessed on May 1, 2022.
19. National Center for Health Statistics (US). Health, United States, 2014: with special feature on adults aged 55–64. Hyattsville, MD: National Center for Health Statistics (US); 2015. Available from. https://www.ncbi.nlm.nih.gov/books.NBK299348/. Accessed May 1, 2022.

20. Levy B, Paulozzi L, Mack KA, et al. Trends in opioid analgesic-prescribing rates by specialty, U.S., 2007-2012. Am J Prev Med 2015;49(3):409–13.
21. Hoffman EM, Watson JC, St Sauver J, et al. Association of long-term opioid therapy with functional status, adverse outcomes, and mortality among patients with polyneuropathy. JAMA Neurol 2017;74(7):773–9.
22. Chou R, Turner JA, Devine EB, et al. The effectiveness and risks of long-term opioid therapy for chronic pain: a systematic review for a national institutes of health pathways to prevention workshop. Ann Inter Med 2015;162(4):276–86.
23. Dowell D, Haegerich TM, Chou R. CDC guidelines for prescribing opioids for chronic pain – United States, 2016. MMWR Recomm Rep 2016;65(1):1–49.
24. Dowell D, Haegerich T, Chou R. No shortcuts to safer opioid prescribing. N Engl J Med 2019;380:2285–7.
25. Kroenke K, Alford DP, Argoff C, et al. Challenges with implementing the centers for disease control and prevention opioid guideline: a consensus panel report. Pain Med 2019;20:724–35.
26. Kertesz SG, Gordon AJ. A crisis of opioids and the limits of prescription control: United States. Addiction 2019;114(1):169–80.
27. Regulations.gov. Proposed 2022 CDC clinical practice guidelines for prescribing opioids. Available at: https://www.regulations.gov/docket/CDC-2022-0024/comments. Accessed May 22, 2022.
28. Reuben DB, Alvanzo AA, Ashikaga T, et al. National institutes of health pathways to prevention workshop: the role of opioids in the treatment of chronic pain. Ann Intern Med 2015;162(4):295–300.
29. Kroenke K, Cheville A. Management of chronic pain in the aftermath of the opioid backlash. JAMA 2017;317(23):2365–6.
30. US Dept of Health and Human Services. HHS guide for clinicians on the appropriate dosage reduction or discontinuation of long-term opioid analgesics. 2019. Available at: https://www.hhs.gov/opioids/sites/default/files/2019-10/Dosage_Reduction_Discontinuation.pdf. Accessed April 15, 2022.
31. Henry SG, Paterniti DA, Feng B, et al. Patients' experience with opioid tapering: a conceptual model with recommendations for clinicians. J Pain 2019;20(2):181–91.
32. Frank JW, Levy C, Matlock DD, et al. Patients' perspectives on tapering of chronic opioid therapy: a qualitative study. Pain Med 2016;17(10):1838–47.
33. Agnoli A, Xing G, Tancredi DJ, et al. Association of dose tapering with overdose or mental health crisis among patients prescribed long-term opioids. JAMA 2021;326(5):411–9 [published correction appears in JAMA. 2022 Feb 15;327(7):688] [published correction appears in JAMA. 2022 Feb 15;327(7):687].
34. U.S. Food and Drug Administration. FDA identifies harm reported from sudden discontinuation of opioid pain medicines and requires label changes to guide prescribers on gradual, individualized tapering: FDA Drug Safety Communication. 2019. Available at: https://www.fda.gov/drugs/drug-safety-and-availability/fda-identifies-harm-reported-sudden-discontinuation-opioid-pain-medicines-and-requires-label-changes. Accessed May 31, 2022.
35. James JR, Scott JM, Klein JW, et al. Mortality after discontinuation of primary care-based chronic opioid therapy for pain: a retrospective cohort study. J Gen Intern Med 2019;34(12):2749–55.
36. Demidenko MI, Dobscha SK, Morasco BJ, et al. Suicidal ideation and suicidal self-directed violence following clinician-initiated prescription opioid discontinuation among long-term opioid users. Gen Hosp Psychiatry 2017;47:29–35.

37. Oliva EM, Bowe T, Manhapra A, et al. Associations between stopping prescriptions for opioids, length of opioid treatment, and overdose or suicide deaths in US veterans: observational evaluation. BMJ 2020;368:m283.
38. Morphine (systemic). Lexi-drugs. Hudson, OH: Lexicomp; 2022. Available at: http://online.lexi.com/. Accessed May 27, 2022.
39. Acetaminophen and codeine. Lexi-Drugs. Hudson, OH: Lexicomp; 2022. Available at: http://online.lexi.com/. Accessed May 27, 2022.
40. Hydrocodone and acetaminophen. Lexi-drugs. Hudson, OH: Lexicomp; 2022. Available at: http://online.lexi.com/. Accessed May 27, 2022.
41. OxyCODONE. Lexi-drugs. Hudson, OH: Lexicomp; 2022. Available at: http://online.lexi.com/. Accessed May 27, 2022.
42. HYDROmorphone lexi-drugs. Hudson, OH: Lexicomp; 2022. Available at: http://online.lexi.com/. Accessed May 27, 2022.
43. DULoxetine. Lexi-Drugs. Hudson, OH: Lexicomp; 2022. Available at: http://online.lexi.com/. Accessed May 27, 2022.
44. Gabapentin. Lexi-drugs. Hudson, OH: Lexicomp; 2022. Available at: http://online.lexi.com/. Accessed May 27, 2022.
45. Pregabalin. Lexi-drugs. Hudson, OH: Lexicomp; 2022. Available at: http://online.lexi.com/. Accessed May 27, 2022.

ADDITIONAL RESOURCES

MME calculator is embedded in the CDC opioid guidelines mobile app that you can download here. Available at: https://www.cdc.gov/drugoverdose/prescribing/app.html.

Tapering Opioids for Chronic Pain (4min 16 sec video). Available at: https://www.cdc.gov/opioids/providers/prescribing/videos.html.

Pocket Guide: Tapering Opioids for Chronic Pain from the CDC. Available at: https://www.cdc.gov/drugoverdose/pdf/clinical_pocket_guide_tapering-a.pdf.

HHS. Opioid Epidemic by the Numbers Infographic. Available at: https://www.hhs.gov/opioids/sites/default/files/2021-02/opioids-infographic.pdf.

NIDA. Opioid Crisis and Pain Management website. Available at: https://nida.nih.gov/nidamed-medical-health-professionals/opioid-crisis-pain-management.

Medications for the Gut

Sean Smithgall, PharmD, BCACP

KEYWORDS

• Gastroesophageal reflux disease • Constipation • Diarrhea • Proton-pump inhibitors • Antacids • Probiotics

KEY POINTS

- Proton-pump inhibitors are the most potent medication for gastroesophageal reflux disease and take up to 5 days for full effect.
- First-line treatment for constipation is increasing dietary fiber.
- Diarrhea is often caused by infectious pathogens and medications should be reserved for select cases.
- Probiotics have questionable benefits for several gut-related disorders and are generally found to be safe to use.

INTRODUCTION

Medications are used in gastrointestinal (GI) disorders to modify gastric pH, heal ulcerations, change intestinal motility, and change gastric secretions. Many medication classes have functionality in different GI disorders including proton-pump inhibitors (PPIs) and dietary fiber. This article explores common medications used in gastroesophageal reflux disease (GERD), constipation, diarrhea, and peptic-ulcer disease (PUD). This article also overviews the use of probiotics in GI conditions. The focus of this article is on the general management of GI conditions and does not include advanced management of rare and complex GI disorders.

GASTRO-ESOPHAGEAL REFLUX DISEASE TREATMENT

Antacids, histamine-2 receptor antagonists (H2Ras), and PPIs are the three primary medication classes used in GERD for anti-reflux. Each class has a different onset of action, duration, and overall potency requiring individualized therapy for each patient. With the exception of cimetidine, the within class medications are equally efficacious and can be interchanged as needed.[1,2] **Table 1** shows which medications are available over-the-counter (OTC). Some PPIs and H2RAs can be prescribed at higher doses than OTC. Each class will be discussed with brief mention of medications with questionable benefits or circumstantial use.

Auburn University Harrison College of Pharmacy, 650 Clinic Drive, Suite 2100, Mobile, AL 36688, USA
E-mail address: Ses0131@auburn.edu

Physician Assist Clin 8 (2023) 339–351
https://doi.org/10.1016/j.cpha.2022.10.011

Table 1
Over-the-counter anti-reflux medications[20]

Class	Medication Brand	Generic/Ingredients	Strength	Formulations	Quantity (Price)[a]
Proton-pump inhibitors (PPIs)	Nexium®	Esomeprazole	20 mg	Capsules	42 ($14.97)
	Prilosec®	Omeprazole	20 mg	Capsules	42 ($14.97)
	Prevacid®	Lansoprazole	15 mg	Capsules	42 ($13.12)
	Zegerid®	Omeprazole Sodium bicarbonate	20 mg 1100 mg	Capsules	42 ($22.84)
H2 receptor antagonists (H2RAs)	Pepcid®	Famotidine	10 mg 20 mg	Tabs	90 ($7.88) 50 ($4.98)
	Zantac®[b]	Ranitidine	75 mg 150 mg	Off market	Off market
	Tagamet®	Cimetidine	200 mg	Tabs	60 ($4.98)
	Zantac 360®	Famotidine	10 mg 20 mg	Tabs	25 ($8.82)
Antacids	Tums®	Calcium carbonate	REG 500 mg EXT 750 mg ULT 1000 mg	Chewable tabs Chewy bites Smooth dissolve	REG 150 ($7.19) EXT 96 ($3.97) ULT 160 ($3.82)
	Tums with Gas Relief®	Calcium carbonate Simethicone	750 mg 80 mg	Chewy bites	28 ($3.97)
	Rolaids® *Regular (Ultra) strength*	Magnesium hydroxide Calcium carbonate	45 (200) mg 220 (1000) mg	Chewable tabs Soft chews	REG 150 ($7.20) EXT 96 ($3.99) ULT 72 ($6.09)
	Rolaids Advanced®	Magnesium hydroxide Calcium carbonate Simethicone	200 mg 1000 mg 40 mg	Chewable tabs Soft chews	60 ($3.84) 28 ($5.39)
	Gaviscon® Regular (Extra) strength	Aluminum hydroxide Magnesium trisilicate (extra contains magnesium carbonate) Alginic acid	80 (160) mg 14.2 (105) mg	Chewable tabs Liquid	100 ($11.16) 12 oz ($8.37)

(*continued on next page*)

Table 1
(continued)

Class	Medication Brand	Generic/Ingredients	Strength	Formulations	Quantity (Price)[a]
	Mylanta®	Aluminum hydroxide Magnesium hydroxide Simethicone[c]	800 mg/10 mL 800 mg/10 mL 80 mg/10 mL	Liquid Chews	12 oz ($6.97) 50 ($8.54)
	Alka-Seltzer®	Anhydrous citric acid Aspirin Sodium bicarbonate	1000 mg 325 mg 1916 mg	Effervescent tablets	72 ($8.42)

Abbreviations: EXT, extra strength; REG, regular strength; ULT, ultra-strength.
[a] Pricing per Walmart ecommerce storefront and are a mix of brand and generic prices. Brand products are more expensive to equivalent generic quantities.
[b] Recalled, no longer available as of 2020.
[c] Simethicone only available in chews.

Antacids

Antacids have the fastest onset of action and shortest duration and therefore are best taken as needed for immediate relief.[3,4] Antacids are also the least potent of the anti-reflux classes and are available as single or combination products containing calcium, aluminum, magnesium, or sodium bicarbonate.[3,4] The elemental metal directly binds protons in the stomach increasing the pH within minutes of administration.[5] However, once the antacid is digested, it is no longer able to bind free protons and ceases to work.[5] This entire process of administration and digestion takes 1 to 3 h giving antacids an overall duration of effect of approximately 2 h.[3]

Antacids come in different formulations including chewable tablets, liquid, and effervescent tablets (see **Table 1**), are well tolerated and have minimal adverse drug reactions (ADR). The most common ADRs include constipation with products containing calcium or aluminum and diarrhea with products that contain magnesium.[4] Aluminum and magnesium are purposefully combined to neutralize the constipation and diarrhea adverse effects. Many products contain the antiflatulent simethicone to decrease the surface tension of gas bubbles and can be useful when bloating is a concomitant symptom. Antacids have the potential to chelate to certain drugs, like azole antifungals, when administered simultaneously and should be separated by 2 h from antacid administration.[6]

Alginic acid, or alginate, forms a raft-like substance that floats on top of gastric contents creating a physical barrier and preventing gastric contents from refluxing through the esophagus.[7] When administered with an antacid, the alginic acid also synergizes with the effects of the antacid by concentrating the antacid underneath the raft.[3] Alginic acid is an inactive ingredient and will only show up under the inactive ingredient list on the medication packaging. Antacids formations with alginate were found to be more effective than those without.[7]

Histamine-2 Receptor Antagonists

H2RAs have a quick onset of action, medium duration of action, and contain characteristics of both antacids and proton pump inhibitors.[8] H2RAs work within 30 min allowing them to be taken as needed for symptoms relief while also having a duration of action of around 8 to 12 h which allows daily administration for chronic GERD.[3,4,8] H2RAs work by inhibiting histamin-2 receptors on the basal membrane of parietal cells eventually blocking some activation of proton pumps.[8] As proton pumps are also activated by acetylcholine and gastrin, H2RAs only block one-third of the activators compared with PPIs which directly block the proton pump.[9] The partial blocking of proton pumps with H2RAs leads to this class being more potent than antacids, but less potent than PPIs.[10]

Famotidine and cimetidine are the most prescribed H2RAs and are also available OTC. Ranitidine was a popular H2RAs until it was recalled in 2020 for containing cancer-causing N-Nitrosodimethylamine (NDMA).[11] Ranitidine is still not available with no news of a future release. Makers of Zantac released a new product in 2021 called Zantac 360 which contains generic famotidine and appears to be no different than the brand name Pepcid.[8] Cimetidine is used less often than famotidine because it is also a potent inhibitor of cytochrome P450 (CYP450) leading to increased concentrations of certain anticoagulants, anti-epileptics, and cardiovascular medications.[8,12–14]

H2RAs are well tolerated in children, adolescents, and adults. H2RAs are cleared by the kidneys and can accumulate in patients with chronic kidney disease.[8] Older adults, age 60 and older, are at risk of having altered mental status (agitation, confusion, and delirium) when taking H2RAs and this effect is compounded in kidney disease, therefore, these medications should be avoided in this patient population.[8]

Proton-Pump Inhibitors

PPIs are the most potent anti-reflux medications available because they irreversibly bind to active proton pumps.[9,10,15] Approximately 70% are active at a given time and pumps are most active before the first meal of the day.[15] With the exception of dexlansoprazole, all PPIs should be given 30 to 60 min before the first meal of the day to allow for maximal binding.[16] Dexlansoprazole has a unique formulation that allows for an extended half-life and can be given regardless of meals.[16] The parietal cells constantly make new pumps, so it takes about 3 to 5 days for PPIs to bind most of the active pumps and reach their full effect.[15]

Length of therapy for PPIs depends on the condition being treated.[2] PPIs are first-line therapy for patients with GERD who also have erosive or nonerosive esophagitis.[2] The treatment of esophagitis is a PPI for 8 weeks.[2] Patients who are not high risk and not actively being treated for esophagitis should be considered for deprescribing of PPI therapy.[2,17] PPIs can either be discontinued or de-escalated to lower doses or H2RA therapy before deprescribing with only 1 in 10 patients having rebound reflux upon discontinuation.[17]

There is a significant amount of clinical controversy over the safety profile of PPIs. PPIs are speculated to decrease nutrient absorption and increase pathogenic bacteria in the gut because of increased gastric pH. Several low-quality studies have shown major ADRs including, but not limited to, myocardial infarction, osteoporosis, fractures, pneumonia, chronic kidney disease, dementia, and clostridium difficile infections.[18] The COMPASS study, a 3-year, prospective, randomized controlled trial evaluating the safety of PPIs showed no significant increase in any of the previously mentioned ADRs and a significant, but rare increase in enteric infections.[19] The COMPASS study was not long enough to rule out some safety concerns with long-term PPI use, but we know that these medications are relatively safe when used for short durations.

Medications with Questionable Benefit in Gastroesophageal Reflux Disease

Baclofen has some use in patients with refractory GERD, but should not be used over other anti-reflux medications.[2] Sucralfate is limited to use during pregnancy due to the localized effect in the gut and the fact that it is not absorbed reducing the harm to the fetus.[2] Pro-kinetics like metoclopramide and erythromycin do not have any use in GERD outside more complex patients with concomitant gastroparesis.[2]

CONSTIPATION TREATMENT

Laxatives are the primary medications used for both acute and chronic forms of constipation and range in mechanisms of action from agents that hydrate and soften stools to agents that stimulate peristalsis to push stool through the gastrointestinal tract (GIT). In addition to laxatives, enemas and suppositories can be used for constipation that has progressed to fecal impaction. Effectiveness of individual agents varies based on dose and route of administration.

Stool Softeners and Bulking Agents

Stool-softeners, or emollients, and bulking agents will hydrate and soften feces over 12 to 72 h.[21,22] Bulk-forming agents, also known as dietary fiber, include methylcellulose, polycarbophil, and psyllium.[21,22] A systematic review showed psyllium is the most effective dietary fiber across all age groups.[23] Dietary fiber increases the size and water content in stools making them easier to pass.[21,22] Patients should be instructed to drink plenty of water while taking fiber to prevent worsened constipation or obstruction. Patients without an underlying condition contributing to the constipation will improve or fully treat the constipation 85% of the time using dietary fiber.[24] Most older adults who increase dietary fiber intake can discontinue other forms of laxatives.[24] Emollients act as surfactants and improve water absorption with the most common being docusate sodium.[21] Emollients do not induce peristalsis and should not be used as monotherapy for constipation.[22]

Osmotic Laxatives

Osmotic laxatives, including polyethylene glycol (PEG) 3350, lactulose, sorbitol, and magnesium citrate, are non-absorbed substances that increase water transit into the gut by increasing osmotic pressure.[21,22] These cause a bowel movement within 24 to 48 h. PEG 3350 can be taken in low doses (17 g) daily or twice daily as an emollient or in high doses (4 L) as a bowel prep evacuator before colonoscopy.[21,22] Lactulose is less effective than PEG 3350 with more adverse effects, so it is reserved for use in patients with hepatic encephalopathy to increase excretion of ammonia through the feces.[21,22] Sorbitol has a similar mechanism of action and efficacy to lactulose.[21,22] Magnesium citrate works within 30 min to 6 h and is typically reserved for combination with high dose PEG3350 for bowel prep before colonoscopy.[21,22]

Stimulant Laxatives

Stimulant laxatives work by stimulating peristalsis activity on the intestine resulting in increased motility in the gut and a bowel movement in 6 to 12 h.[22] Stimulant laxatives work well when paired with stool softeners due to the complimentary mechanisms of action. About half of patients will get abdominal pain and diarrhea within the first week, but because long-term data beyond 4 weeks is limited, stimulant laxatives should only be used in chronic constipation after first trying dietary fiber or osmotic laxatives.[21,24]

Other Agents

Other medications for chronic constipation include lubiprostone, linaclotide, plecanatide, and prucalopride (**Table 2** for place in therapy).[25] Lubiprostone is a chloride

Table 2
Treatment of acute and chronic constipation[21,23,24]

	Class
Acute (Episodic)	
First-line	Bulking agents (dietary Fiber)
Second-line	Osmotic laxatives
Third-line	Stimulant laxatives with stool softeners
Last-line	Magnesium citrate, bisacodyl rectal, enemas.
Chronic	
First-line	Bulking agents (dietary Fiber) and osmotic laxitives[a]
Second-line	Stimulant laxatives[b]
Last-line	Lubiprostone, linaclotide, plecanatide, and prucalopride

[a] PEG 3350 preferred over other osmotic laxatives.
[b] Bisacodyl most studied agent.

channel activator that improves intestinal fluid secretion and works within 24 h.[21] Linaclotide and plecanatide increase intestinal fluid and GI transit through increased chloride and bicarbonate secretion into the intestines and can take up to a week to start working.[25] Prucalopride is the newest agent and has a unique mechanism agonizing 5-HT_4 receptors increasing peristalsis and secretions in the intestines.[25]

Enemas and Suppositories

Warm water and mineral enemas are useful in patients with fecal impaction and are preferred over phosphate and soapsuds enemas. A safe alternative to enemas is glycerin suppositories.[21] Some hospital systems will have special formulations of enemas like SMOG which stands for saline, mineral oil, and glycerin that are compounded in-house by the pharmacy department at specific ratios.

Safety

Stool softeners and PEG 3350 are the best tolerated and have the least adverse effects. The most common ADRs seen across all laxatives are bloating, nausea, and diarrhea in about 10% of patients. Bisacodyl has the highest rates of diarrhea and abdominal pain at a rate of 56% during week 1 that improves significantly by week 4.[21]

DIARRHEA TREATMENT

Diarrhea is a common condition that can be acute (lasting <14 days), persistent (lasting 14 to 30 days), or chronic (lasting more than 30 days).[26] Acute infectious diarrhea is often self-limiting and the treatment is supportive care with fluids and electrolytes.[26] Taking an anti-diarrheal agent for infectious diarrhea can be dangerous and prevent passage of the invading gut pathogen.[26] Non-infectious acute diarrhea or chronic diarrhea may require medication management, especially in patients with irritable bowel syndrome (IBS) with partial or complete symptoms of diarrhea.

Opiates and Derivatives

Loperamide is an opiate that binds peripherally to inhibit peristalsis, increase anal sphincter tone, and prolongs transit time.[27] As an opiate that crosses the blood–brain barrier, there is an abuse potential when loperamide is given in high doses.[27] In 2016, the Food and Drug Administration (FDA) warned about serious heart problems with high-dose loperamide.[28] Some formulations also contain simethicone.[27]

Diphenoxylate and its metabolite, difenoxin, inhibit excessive GI motility and GI propulsion within 48 h to lessen diarrhea.[27] If no benefit is seen within 48 h, difenoxin should be discontinued.[27] Diphenoxylate can be taken up to 10 days to show a benefit, afterward it should also be discontinued if there is no perceived benefit.[27] Both diphenoxylate and difenoxin are combined with subtherapeutic doses of atropine to prevent abuse.[27] Atropine can cause the potential for anticholinergic ADR like dry mouth, tachycardia, decreased urination, and altered mental status.[27]

Other forms of opioids include paregoric and opium tincture.[27] Paregoric goes through intermittent discontinuation and as of this publication, is currently unavailable in the United States.[27] Paregoric should not be confused with opium tincture, which is 25 times more potent and often reserved for neonatal abstinence syndrome.[27] Opium tincture and paregoric are rarely used for diarrhea due to their abuse potential.[27]

Absorbents and Antisecretory Agents

Bismuth subsalicylate is an antisecretory, anti-inflammatory, and anti-bacterial agent.[27] Depending on the cause of the diarrhea, bismuth subsalicylate can have multiple mechanisms for improving symptoms.[27] Bismuth subsalicylate should be avoided in children less than 18 years of age with viral illnesses like influenza or varicella as this can cause Reye syndrome.[27] Notable ADRs of bismuth include darkened stools and black tongue.[27] Dietary fibers, including polycarbophil and psyllium can also be beneficial in diarrhea due to their absorption effects.[27] Polycarbophil can absorb 60 to 70 times its weight in water and caution should be used if administering with too much water as this can cause choking.[29]

Miscellaneous Agents for Diarrhea

Probiotics are often used for diarrhea on the assumption that strengthening normal flora concentrations will improve symptoms; however, there is limited evidence of benefit and their use is currently not recommended.[26] Specific vaccines are available for travelers who are at risk for cholera.[27] Rifaximin is an antibiotic with low-quality evidence for the treatment of IBS that is diarrhea dominate.[27] Rifaximin should be reserved for when other therapies like dietary fiber and loperamide have failed.[27]

PEPTIC ULCER DISEASE TREATMENT

The three most common types of PUD are as follows: *Helicobacter pylori* induced, nonsteroidal anti-inflammatory drugs (NSAID) induced, or stress-related mucosal damage (SRMD). SRMD occurs in critical care situations and carries a high mortality rate. Patients with trauma, burns, or other critical illnesses, receive prophylactic PPI therapy when admitted to intensive care units to prevent SRMD. Once the critical care situation resolves, the PPI can be discontinued unless there is another reason for PPI use (eg, GERD). NSAID-induced ulcer, most commonly a gastric ulcer, is treated by discontinuing the NSAID and treating with PPI therapy. Based on the severity of NSAID-induced PUD, the patient will receive intravenous or high-dose oral PPI therapy followed by chronic PPI therapy. Following endoscopy, a regimen of high dose intravenous PPI for 72 h followed by twice daily PPI through day 14 showed significantly less re-bleeding and mortality.[30,31]

Helicobacter pylori-induced PUD commonly presents as ulceration in the duodenum.[33] Because treatment of *H pylori* requires a combination of antibiotics, PPI, and sometimes bismuth subsalicylate, it is important to test for its presence anytime PUD is suspected.[33] PPIs can interfere with testing of *H pylori* PUD and should be held 2 weeks before rapid urease testing and urea breath testing.[33] Bismuth salts should be held 4 weeks before rapid urease testing, or another test should be selected.[33] When testing for eradication, wait 4 weeks after antibiotics and 2 weeks after PPI use to prevent suppression of *H pylori* and the potential for false negatives.[33] According to recent guidelines, all multi-drug regimens for *H pylori* are considered first-line; however, bismuth quadruple therapy and non-bismuth quadruple therapy have stronger evidence to support their benefit (**Table 3** lists regimens).[33] Regimens with clarithromycin should be avoided when local resistance rates are 15% or greater.[33]

Table 3
Regimens for the treatment of *Helicobacter pylori* peptic-ulcer disease[33]

Regimen	Duration (Days)	Drug 1	Drug 2	Drug 3	Drug 4
Bismuth quadruple[a]	10 to 14	PPI or H2RA Daily or BID	Bismuth subsalicylate 525 mg QID	Metronidazole 250 to 500 mg QID	Tetracycline 500 mg QID
Non-bismuth Quadruple[a]	10 to 14	PPI Daily or BID	Clarithromycin 250 to 500 mg BID	Amoxicillin 1 g BID	Metronidazole 250 to 500 mg BID
PPI triple[b]	14	PPI daily or BID Daily or BID	Clarithromycin 500 mg BID	Amoxicillin 1 g BID or Metronidazole 500 mg BID	
Sequential	10	PPI Daily or BID Days 1 to 10	Amoxicillin 1 g BID Days 1 to 5	Metronidazole 250 to 500 mg BID Days 6 to 10	Clarithromycin 250 to 500 mg BID Days 6 to 10
Hybrid	14	PPI Daily or BID Days 1 to 14	Amoxicillin 1 g BID Days 1 to 14	Metronidazole 250 to 500 mg BID Days 7 to 14	Clarithromycin 250 to 500 mg BID Days 7 to 14
Levofloxacin triple	10 to 14	PPI BID	Levofloxacin 500 mg daily	Amoxicillin 1 g BID	
Levofloxacin sequential	10	PPI BID Days 1 to 10	Amoxicillin 1 g BID Days 1 to 10	Levofloxacin 500 mg daily Days 6 to 10	Metronidazole 500 mg BID Days 6 to 10
LOAD	7 to 10	PPI Daily (high dose)	Levofloxacin 250 mg daily	Nitazoxanide (Alinia®)[c] 500 mg BID	Doxycycline 100 mg daily

Abbreviations: BID, twice daily; H2RA, histamine-2 receptor agonist; LOAD, levofloxacin; omeprazole, Alinia; and doxycycline; PPI, proton-pump inhibitor; QID, four-times daily.

[a] Strong recommendation.
[b] No longer recommended due to resistance rates.
[c] Expensive medication which limits the use of LOAD therapy over other cheaper alternatives

Data from 2011 show the resistance rate of clarithromycin in *H pylori* was 16% in the United States.[33]

BENEFITS OF PROBIOTICS

Probiotics can be prescribed or purchased OTC and differ significantly from one product to the next. Probiotics contain bacteria or other microorganisms that reflect the natural bacteria, or normal flora, found within the GIT.[34] It is logical that these microorganisms would have a role in gut health given their similarity to normal flora and they are often used for suppression of growth of pathogenic bacteria, improvement of intestinal barrier function, modulation of the immune system, and modulation of pain perception.[35] About 20% of adults use a daily probiotic to promote healthy digestion and bowel habits.[34] Popularity for probiotics continues to grow each year with estimated market sales of approximately 62 billion in 2022 with forecasted growth of approximately 110 billion by 2030.[36] The most common species within probiotics are *Lactobacillus*, *Bifidobacterium*, or *Saccharomyces*.[34] There are numerous subspecies of bacteria with each manufactured product being slightly different making it difficult to evaluate the true benefit of probiotics.

Clinical Pearls with Probiotics

- Target dose is 5 billion colony-forming units per day.[37]
- Probiotic benefit of yogurt containing live cultures is controversial as potential for breakdown by stomach acid is greater for yogurt than supplements.[32]
- No benefit for probiotics in children with diarrhea and conflicting evidence for adults with diarrhea.[35]
- May benefit inflammatory bowel disease, but guideline-directed therapy should still be used first.
- Systematic review and meta-analysis showed no benefit for probiotics in preventing or treating antibiotic-associated diarrhea.[38]
- Meta-analysis showed no benefit in *H pylori* eradication with probiotics.[39]
- Small randomized-controlled trials showed efficacy for probiotics in treating general constipation and infrequent bowel habits.[40,41]
- Among 387 studies, probiotics were well tolerated with no significant increase in adverse drug reactions.[38]
- Caution when using in patients who are immunocompromised as probiotics could lead to bacteremia or fungemia.[38]

Despite the lack of efficacy, patients who are taking probiotics and believe they are helping them should not be pushed to discontinue the products as they are generally safe.

SUMMARY

Medications for the gut have different mechanisms of action and efficacy for each GI indication. GERD treatment should be individualized to the patient with PPI reserved for patients with esophagitis, or severe symptoms. Constipation is best prevented with dietary fiber; however, there are more potent agents for immediate evacuation. Diarrhea has not been shown to be prevented with probiotics and opioid-like drugs are the most effective treatment despite their abuse potential. PUD regimens can be complex and require careful consideration of local resistance rates. Probiotics in general may or may not have benefits in certain conditions; however, they are overall safe, and patients should be fine taking them.

CLINICS CARE POINTS

- Proton-Pump Inhibitors are the most potent anti-reflux medication, are more expensive than other options, and have been shown to be relatively safe.
- Dietary fiber is a safe and effective option for both diarrhea and constipation.
- Treatment of *H. pylori* peptic ulcer disease requires adherence to multi-drug, two-week regimens and evaluation of local bacterial resistance rates.
- Porbiotics are popular for gut-related disorders despite a lack of quality evidence showing the benefit of specific products.

DISCLOSURE

The author has no conflicts to disclose.

REFERENCES

1. Merki HS, Witzel L, Walt RP, et al. Double blind comparison of the effects of cimetidine, ranitidine, famotidine, and placebo on intragastric acidity in 30 normal volunteers. Gut 1988;29(1):81–4.
2. Katz PO, Dunbar KB, Schnoll-Sussman FH, et al. ACG clinical guideline for the diagnosis and management of gastroesophageal reflux disease. Am J Gastroenterol 2022;117(1):27–56. https://doi.org/10.14309/ajg.0000000000001538.
3. MacFarlane B. Management of gastroesophageal reflux disease in adults: a pharmacist's perspective. Integr Pharm Res Pract 2018;7:41–52.
4. Savarino E, Zentilin P, Marabotto E, et al. A review of pharmacotherapy for treating gastroesophageal reflux disease (GERD). Expert Opin Pharmacother 2017; 18(13):1333–43.
5. Heller HJ, Stewart A, Haynes S, et al. Pharmacokinetics of calcium absorption from two commercial calcium supplements. J Clin Pharmacol 1999;39(11): 1151–4.
6. Calcium carbonate, aluminum hydroxide, magnesium hydroxide. Lexi-drugs. Hudson, OH: Lexicomp; 2022. Available at: http://online.lexi.com/. Accessed April 25, 2022.
7. Leiman DA, Riff BP, Morgan S, et al. Alginate therapy is effective treatment for GERD symptoms: a systematic review and meta-analysis. Dis Esophagus 2017;30(5):1–9.
8. Famotidine, cimetidine. Lexi-drugs. Hudson, OH: Lexicomp; 2022. Available at: http://online.lexi.com/. Accessed April 30, 2022.
9. Helander HF. Physiology and pharmacology of the parietal cell. Baillieres Clin Gastroenterol 1988;2(3):539–54.
10. Wang W-H, Huang J-Q, Zheng G-F, et al. Head-to-head comparison of H2-receptor antagonists and proton pump inhibitors in the treatment of erosive esophagitis: a meta-analysis. World J Gastroenterol 2005;11(26):4067–77.
11. FDA Requests Removal of All Ranitidine Products (Zantac) from the Market [press release]. 2020. Available at: https://www.fda.gov/news-events/press-

announcements/fda-requests-removal-all-ranitidine-products-zantac-market. Accessed June 22, 2022.
12. Sabesin SM. Safety issues relating to long-term treatment with histamine H2-receptor antagonists. Aliment Pharmacol Ther 1993;7(Suppl 2):35–40.
13. Carroll DN, Carroll DG. Interactions between warfarin and three commonly prescribed fluoroquinolones. Ann Pharmacother 2008;42(5):680–5.
14. Pino MA, Azer SA. Cimetidine. In: StatPearls. Treasure island (FL): StatPearls Publishing LLC.; 2022. StatPearls Publishing Copyright © 2022.
15. Shin JM, Sachs G. Pharmacology of proton pump inhibitors. Curr Gastroenterol Rep 2008;10(6):528–34.
16. Dexlansoprazole. Lexi-drugs. Hudson, OH: Lexicomp; 2022. Available at: http://online.lexi.com/. Accessed April 25, 2022.
17. Farrell B, Pottie K, Thompson W, et al. Deprescribing proton pump inhibitors. Evidence-based clinical practice guideline. Can Fam Physician 2017;63(5):354–64.
18. Yadlapati R, Kahrilas PJ. When is proton pump inhibitor use appropriate? BMC Med 2017;15(1):36.
19. Moayyedi P, Eikelboom JW, Bosch J, et al. Safety of Proton Pump Inhibitors Based on a Large, Multi-Year, Randomized Trial of Patients Receiving Rivaroxaban or Aspirin. Gastroenterology 2019;157(3):682–91, e682.
20. Pharmacy, Health, and Wellness. Walmart. Available at: https://www.walmart.com/. Accessed April, 2022.
21. Mounsey A, Raleigh M, Wilson A. Management of Constipation in Older Adults. Am Fam Physician 2015;92(6):500–4.
22. Laxatives. Lexi-drugs. Hudson, OH: Lexicomp; 2022. Available at: http://online.lexi.com/. Accessed April 25, 2022.
23. Suares NC, Ford AC. Systematic review: the effects of fibre in the management of chronic idiopathic constipation. Aliment Pharmacol Ther 2011;33(8):895–901.
24. Paquette IM, Varma M, Ternent C, et al. The American Society of Colon and Rectal Surgeons' Clinical Practice Guideline for the Evaluation and Management of Constipation. Dis Colon Rectum 2016;59(6):479–92.
25. Lubiprostone, linaclotide, plecanatide, prucalopride. Lexi-Drugs. Hudson, OH: Lexicomp; 2022. Available at: http://online.lexi.com/. Accessed April 25, 2022.
26. Riddle MS, DuPont HL, Connor BA. ACG Clinical Guideline: Diagnosis, Treatment, and Prevention of Acute Diarrheal Infections in Adults. Am J Gastroenterol 2016;111(5):602–22.
27. Antidiarrheals Lexi-Drugs. Hudson, OH: Lexicomp; 2022. Available at: http://online.lexi.com/. Accessed April 25, 2022.
28. FDA Drug Safety Communication. FDA warns about serious heart problems with high doses of the antidiarrheal medicine loperamide (Immodium), including from abuse and misuse. [press release]. 2016. Available at: https://www.fda.gov/drugs/drug-safety-and-availability/fda-drug-safety-communication-fda-warns-about-serious-heart-problems-high-doses-antidiarrheal. Accessed June 22, 2022.
29. Iwanaga Y. [Physicochemical and pharmacological characteristic and clinical efficacy of an anti-irritable bowel syndrome agent, polycarbophil calcium (Polyful)]. Nihon Yakurigaku Zasshi 2002;119(3):185–90.
30. Barkun AN, Almadi M, Kuipers EJ, et al. Management of nonvariceal upper gastrointestinal bleeding: guideline recommendations from the international consensus group. Ann Intern Med 2019;171(11):805–22.
31. Stanley AJ, Laine L. Management of acute upper gastrointestinal bleeding. BMJ 2019;364:l536.

32. Chey WD, Leontiadis GI, Howden CW, et al. ACG clinical guideline: treatment of *Helicobacter pylori* infection. Am J Gastroenterol 2017;112(2):212–39.
33. Pedrosa MC, Golner BB, Goldin BR, et al. Survival of yogurt-containing organisms and Lactobacillus gasseri (ADH) and their effect on bacterial enzyme activity in the gastrointestinal tract of healthy and hypochlorhydric elderly subjects. Am J Clin Nutr 1995;61(2):353–9.
34. Wilkins T, Sequoia J. probiotics for gastrointestinal conditions: a summary of the evidence. Am Fam Physician 2017;96(3):170–8.
35. Preidis GA, Weizman AV, Kashyap PC, et al. AGA technical review on the role of probiotics in the management of gastrointestinal disorders. Gastroenterology 2020;159(2):708–38, e704.
36. Probiotics market size: industry report, 2021-2030. probiotics market size. Available at: https://www.grandviewresearch.com/industry-analysis/probiotics-market. Accessed April 10, 2022.
37. Goldenberg JZ, Lytvyn L, Steurich J, et al. Probiotics for the prevention of pediatric antibiotic-associated diarrhea. Cochrane Database Syst Rev 2015;(12): Cd004827.
38. Hempel S, Newberry SJ, Maher AR, et al. Probiotics for the prevention and treatment of antibiotic-associated diarrhea: a systematic review and meta-analysis. J Am Med Assoc 2012;307(18):1959–69.
39. Lu C, Sang J, He H, et al. Probiotic supplementation does not improve eradication rate of *Helicobacter pylori* infection compared with placebo based on standard therapy: a meta-analysis. Sci Rep 2016;6:23522.
40. Dimidi E, Christodoulides S, Fragkos KC, et al. The effect of probiotics on functional constipation in adults: a systematic review and meta-analysis of randomized controlled trials. Am J Clin Nutr 2014;100(4):1075–84.
41. Miller LE, Ouwehand AC, Ibarra A. Effects of probiotic-containing products on stool frequency and intestinal transit in constipated adults: systematic review and meta-analysis of randomized controlled trials. Ann Gastroenterol 2017; 30(6):629–39.

Medicines for the Kidney

Lavinia Salama, PharmD[a], Steven Sica, PharmD[b],
Katie E. Cardone, PharmD, BCACP, FNKF, FASN, FCCP[c,*]

KEYWORDS

- Medication use • Dosing • Chronic kidney disease (CKD) • Hyperkalemia
- Anemia of CKD • CKD-MBD

KEY POINTS

- Chronic kidney disease (CKD) is progressive and leads to decreased renal filtration, metabolic function, and endocrine functions of the kidney. As CKD progresses, the pharmacokinetics and pharmacodynamics of many medications are altered. Dialysis removal of medications should be considered in patients receiving kidney replacement therapies.
- Angiotensin-converting enzyme inhibitors and angiotensin II receptor blockers are considered first-line agents in the management of proteinuria, hypertension, and slowing down the progression of CKD. Sodium–glucose cotransporter-2 inhibitors can be used to slow the progression of CKD in patients with and without diabetes. The nonsteroidal mineralocorticoid receptor antagonist finerenone is approved to slow CKD progression in patients with diabetes.
- Hyperkalemia treatment varies depending on acuity and severity and may include a combination of medications to stabilize the myocardium, shift potassium intracellularly ("hide" potassium), or eliminate potassium from the body.
- Anemia of CKD is typically treated with a combination of iron supplementation and erythropoietin-stimulating agents to prevent the need for blood transfusions.
- CKD-mineral and bone disease is typically managed through dietary phosphorus restriction, phosphate binders, vitamin D analogs, and calcimimetics.

INTRODUCTION

Patients with altered kidney function have unique medication needs. Medication regimens may require adjustments to the specific medications used, doses, or instructions, ultimately increasing regimen complexity.[1–3] Medication therapy problems lead to frequent hospitalizations and excess burden to the health care system. It is therefore important to identify patients with kidney impairment across care settings, critically evaluate their medication regimens, and adjust as necessary.

[a] University of Wyoming School of Pharmacy, 821 East 18th Street, Cheyenne, WY 82001 USA; [b] Yale New Haven Health, Outpatient Pharmacy Services, 1100 Sherman Avenue, Hamden, CT 06514 USA; [c] Albany College of Pharmacy and Health Sciences, 106 New Scotland Avenue, Albany, NY 12208, USA
* Corresponding author.
E-mail address: katie.cardone@acphs.edu

Physician Assist Clin 8 (2023) 353–369
https://doi.org/10.1016/j.cpha.2022.10.012
physicianassistant.theclinics.com

Kidney impairment is classified as acute kidney injury (AKI), chronic kidney disease (CKD), or acute kidney disease (AKD) as defined in **Fig. 1** and **Tables 1** and **2**.[4–6] In this article, the authors focus on medications used in the treatment of CKD as this disease affects at least one in seven Americans.[7] Medication interventions focus in three areas:

- Preserve kidney function
- Manage complications
- Adjust medications based on kidney function

Preserve Kidney Function

Slowing CKD progression is important as worsening estimated glomerular filtration rate (eGFR) and the presence of albuminuria increase risk for both morbidity and mortality.[4] Strategies include managing underlying conditions contributing to CKD, for example, managing diabetes and blood pressure, smoking cessation, weight loss, and use of specific medication classes, including angiotensin-converting enzyme inhibitors and angiotensin receptor blockers (ACEis/ARBs), sodium-glucose cotransporter-2 inhibitors (SGLT2i), and mineralocorticoid receptor antagonists (MRAs) (particularly finerenone).[4,8–10]

Treating hypertension

Hypertension is a common condition in CKD and is both a cause and complication of the disease. CKD contributes to hypertension through multiple mechanisms including volume overload, sympathetic overactivity, sodium retention, endothelial dysfunction, and potential alterations in blood pressure regulation. The 11,12 KDIGO guidelines recommend a target systolic blood pressure (SBP) less than 120 mm Hg in CKD (using standardized office BP techniques), a less intensive target in limited life expectancy or postural hypotension, and less than 130/80 mm Hg in kidney transplant.[11]

Some lifestyle interventions for hypertension require modification in CKD.[12] Although most patients should limit dietary sodium intake (<2 g/day), sodium restriction may not be appropriate in sodium-wasting nephropathy. For patients with CKD adherence to the Dietary Approach to Stop Hypertension (DASH diet) can result in hyperkalemia due to the high potassium content of the diet.[11,13,14]

Patients with CKD often have resistant or difficult to control hypertension requiring ≥3 antihypertensives. According to the 2021 KDIGO Hypertension guidelines,[11] the use of ACEis or ARBs are first line, particularly when albuminuria is present. On the initiation of these medications, there is a predictable increase in serum creatinine

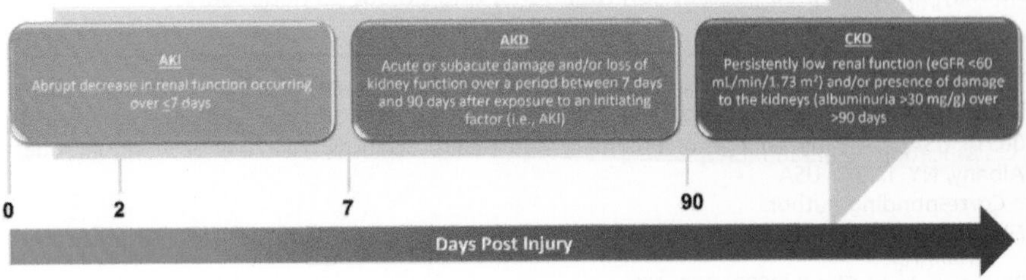

Fig. 1. Definitions of kidney impairment.[31] AKD, acute kidney disease; AKI, acute kidney injury; CKD, chronic kidney disease; eGFR, estimated glomerular filtration rate.

Table 1
Classification of chronic kidney disease by glomerular filtration rate category[4]

GFR Categories (mL/min/1.73 m^2	G1[a]	Normal	≥90
	G2[a]	Mildly decreased	60–89
	G3a	Mildly to moderately decreased	45–59
	G3b	Moderately to severely decreased	30–44
	G4	Severely decreased	15–29
	G5	Kidney failure	<15

[a] Kidney damage present.

(SCr) and a risk for hyperkalemia. Thus, monitoring SCr and potassium (K) within 4 weeks of initiation or dose change is recommended. An SCr increase less than 30% from baseline does not mandate automatic dosage decrease/discontinuation. An Scr increase greater than 30% from baseline warrants investigation for causes such as volume depletion, dehydration, or use of nephrotoxic medications. Hyperkalemia can develop at any point during therapy and can be managed with the use of potassium binders (described later in this article).

Other medications used in the treatment of hypertension are the same as those for patients without concomitant CKD and are discussed in the article, Best Practices in Medical Management of Chronic Hypertension. Historically, thiazide diuretics were stopped when a patient's glomerular filtration rate (GFR) was below 30 mL/min/1.73 m^2. However, the recent CLICK study evaluated the use of chlorthalidone in patients with eGFR 15 to 30 mL/min/1.73 m^2 and hypertension (HTN) control benefit was observed.[15] The steroidal MRAs, spironolactone, and eplerenone reduce blood pressure in resistant hypertension.[16] When added to ACEi/ARB, MRAs may reduce systolic blood pressure and proteinuria.

Treating diabetes

Controlling blood glucose prevents microvascular complications of the disease, including nephropathy.[8] The 2020 KDIGO diabetes guidelines recommend individualized glycated hemoglobin (A1C) based on comorbidities, propensity for hypoglycemia, life expectancy, stage of CKD, and macrovascular complications. The A1C goal ranges from less than 6.5 to less than 8%. These guidelines recommend that patients with diabetes and CKD receive metformin plus an SGLT2 inhibitor as initial therapy. Both therapies are limited as GFR declines with metformin contraindicated at an eGFR less than 30 mL/min/1.73 m^2. For the SGLT2 inhibitors, dapagliflozin and canagliflozin are currently indicated for slowing progression of CKD and decreasing cardiovascular risk. Dapagliflozin can be initiated at an eGFR greater than 25 mL/min/1.73 m^2 and is indicated in patients both with and without diabetes. Canagliflozin can be initiated at an eGFR > 30 mL/min/1.73 m^2 and is indicated in patients with

Table 2
Classification by albuminuria category[4]

Persistent Albuminuria Categories	A1	A2	A3
	Normal to mildly increased	Moderately increased	Severely increased
	<30 mg/g or <3 mg/mmol	30–300 mg/g or 3–30 mg/mmol	>300 mg/g or >30 mg/mmol

diabetes. The use of empagliflozin to slow CKD progression is being studied in the EMPA KIDNEY trial with results forthcoming. Although the effect on blood glucose reduction wanes as CKD advances, patients prescribed SGLT2 inhibitors can remain on them until dialysis is needed for their nephroprotective and cardiovascular benefits.[8]

In patients who are intolerant of metformin or SGLT2 inhibitors or who need additional blood glucose lowering, the KDIGO guidelines recommend the use of long-acting glucagon-like peptide-1 receptor agonists.[8]

The nonsteroidal MRA, finerenone, is a new agent that is FDA-approved to slow CKD progression and decrease cardiovascular (CV) events in patients with T2D.[9,17] Finerenone has minimal effects on lowering blood pressure and avoids the sexual side effects of spironolactone and eplerenone.[18] Hyperkalemia is still a concern and requires monitoring.

Managing Complications of Kidney Impairment

Complications of kidney disease can affect various organ systems. This section focuses on the most common complications of CKD, mineral and bone disorder (MBD), hyperkalemia, and anemia.

Chronic kidney disease -mineral and bone disorder

As GFR declines, hyperparathyroidism occurs due to complex feedback mechanisms involving increased phosphate^{-} retention, increased fibroblast growth factor-23 (FGF-23), decreased calcium and 1,25-dihydroxyvitamin D (1,25$(OH)_2$D) concentrations.[19] This process begins as early as CKD G3a, resulting in high bone turnover. In early CKD, decreased phosphate elimination leads to decreased serum calcium. This leads to increased parathyroid hormone (iPTH) synthesis to increase calcium reabsorption, decrease phosphate reabsorption, and increase calcium mobilization from the bones. FGF-23 is a bone-derived hormone that promotes phosphate excretion and decreased synthesis of 1,25$(OH)_2$D. The 2017 KDIGO guidelines recommend the following targets:

- Serum phosphate toward normal range in CKD G3a-G5D
- Serum calcium to avoid hypercalcemia in CKD G3a-G5D; mild asymptomatic hypocalcemia is permitted.
- PTH has unknown optimal levels for CKD 3a-G5 (non-dialysis) and two to nine times the upper limit of normal (ULN) for CKD G5D.
- Serum 25-hydroxyvitamin D: greater than 30 ng/mL.

Non-pharmacologic interventions are focused mainly on dietary interventions and for dialysis-dependent patients, adherence to the dialysis procedure. Guidelines recommend limiting dietary phosphate to 800 to 1200 mg/day in G3a-G5D. Implementation of this is difficult as phosphorus content is rarely listed on food labels. Dairy and protein are typically high in phosphorus but also necessary for good nutrition, and patients with CKD are often asked to limit sodium and potassium; adding phosphorus to the restrictions increases risk of nonadherence and malnutrition.

Parathyroidectomy is reserved for patients with unresponsive hyperparathyroidism who are adherent to their medications. Risk of "hungry bone syndrome" post-op requires calcium supplementation.

Phosphate binders

These are reserved for "progressive or persistently" elevated serum phosphorus concentration.[19] These agents (**Table 3**) bind phosphorus in the gastrointestinal (GI) tract

Table 3
Phosphate binders[19]

Generic (Brand)	Dosage Form	Advantage(s)	Disadvantage(s)
Calcium carbonate (Tums)	Capsules, tablets, suspension, chewable tablets	• Inexpensive	• Calcium-based binders may lead to vascular calcifications • Contains 40% elemental calcium and may lead to hypercalcemia • High pill burden • GI adverse reaction, constipation
Calcium acetate (PhosLo, PhosLyra)	Capsule, oral solution	• Inexpensive • Less elemental calcium compared with calcium carbonate	• Calcium-based binders may lead to vascular calcifications • Contains 21% elemental calcium and may lead to hypercalcemia • GI adverse reaction, constipation
Aluminum hydroxide (AlternaGel)	Suspension	• Inexpensive	• Long-term use is not recommended due to risk of aluminum toxicity, osteomalacia and encephalopathy • GI adverse reaction, constipation
Lanthanum carbonate (Fosrenol)	Chewable tablets, oral powder	• Low pill burden	• Expensive • Tablet must be chewed or crushed completely • GI adverse reactions, abdominal pain, nausea, constipation
Ferric citrate (Auryxia)	Tablets	• Iron absorbed from GI tract could be used to manage iron deficiency anemia in non-dialysis patients	• Expensive • Avoid in patients with iron overload • GI adverse events like abdominal pain, constipation, diarrhea, nausea, darkening of stools

(*continued on next page*)

Table 3
(continued)

Generic (Brand)	Dosage Form	Advantage(s)	Disadvantage(s)
Sucroferric oxyhydroxide (Velphoro)	Chewable tablets	• Low pill burden • No iron absorption, can be used in patients with iron overload	• Expensive • GI adverse reactions, diarrhea, nausea, darkening of stools
Sevelamer carbonate (Renvela)	Tablets, powder for suspension (packets)	• Lowers low-density lipoprotein (LDL) and raises high-density lipoprotein (HDL) • No systemic absorption from intestinal tract, excreted entirely in feces	• Expensive • High pill burden • May decrease absorption of folic acid and fat-soluble vitamins -GI adverse effects including abdominal pain, nausea, constipation
Sevelamer hydrochloride (Renagel)	Tablets	• Lowers LDL and raises HDL • No systemic absorption from intestinal tract, excreted entirely in feces	• Expensive • Risk of metabolic acidosis • Large pill burden • Impairs the absorption of folic acid and fat-soluble vitamins

and prevent absorption. These should be dosed within 5 to 10 minutes before meals or immediately after meals/snacks. Dosage form is an important consideration; patient preferences should inform selection.

Nutritional vitamin D

Correction of 25-hydroxyvitamin D deficiency (levels <30 ng/mL) can partially correct elevated PTH in CKD. Ergocalciferol (vitamin D2) is derived from plant sources. Cholecalciferol (vitamin D3) is derived from sunlight exposure and animal sources. Either form is hepatically hydroxylated to 25-hydroxyvitamin D (calcifediol) then further hydroxylated by 1α-hydroxylase from the kidneys to 1,25-dihydroxyvitamin D (calcitriol). Generally, recommended repletion is ergocalciferol or cholecalciferol 50,000 international units once weekly for 6 to 12 weeks until stores are replenished then 800 to 2000 international units orally daily thereafter.

A newer prescription-only agent, calcifediol is used for CKD G3–G4 with low vitamin D levels.[20,21] Calcifediol has been suggested to be 2 to 3 times more potent and has higher rates of intestinal absorption than cholecalciferol. Its high cost limits its use.

All these agents can lower iPTH which is desired but can also increase serum calcium and phosphorus.

Activated vitamin D analogs (1,25-dihydroxyvitamin). Vitamin D analogs are often required in patients on dialysis and when PTH levels remain persistently elevated despite treatment of hyperphosphatemia and adequate 25-hydroxyvitamin D stores.[19] Calcitriol, paricalcitol, and doxercalciferol are reserved for CKD G4–G5 with severe progressive hyperparathyroidism. These are available as parenteral or oral formulations. Calcitriol is the pharmacologically active form of 1,25-dihydroxyvitamin D3 and does not require hepatic or renal activation. Paricalcitol and doxercalciferol are active vitamin D2 analogs and thought to cause less hypercalcemia compared with calcitriol.

Calcimimetics. Calcimimetics, cinacalcet and etelcalcetide target the calcium-sensing receptor on the parathyroid gland and increase sensitivity to calcium thereby lowering PTH for patients on dialysis. Both can lower serum calcium and phosphorus levels. Cinacalcet is an oral agent, whereas etelcalcetide is intravenous (IV).

Hyperkalemia

Hyperkalemia occurs due to reduced renal potassium excretion. Patients with CKD often tolerate mild increases in serum K+ (5–5.5 mEq/L).[22] Acutely, hyperkalemia is defined as having serum K+ that is above the ULN, which varies slightly by institution.[23] Hyperkalemia can result from imbalances between potassium intake and renal excretion as well as shifts of potassium redistribution from intracellular to extracellular space. Underlying conditions (heart failure, diabetes, and metabolic acidosis), medications (ACEi, ARBs, MRAs, calcineurin inhibitors, digoxin, potassium supplements, and NSAIDs) and diet (salt substitutes, tomatoes, orange, grapefruit, cooked spinach, potatoes, and bananas) can contribute to hyperkalemia.[24]

Hyperkalemia is classified as mild, moderate, or severe based on serum K+ concentration and presence or absence of EKG changes. When serum K+ concentration is between 5 and 5.9 mEq/L in the absence of EKG changes, it is considered mild hyperkalemia. Moderate hyperkalemia is defined as either having serum K+ 5 to 5.9 mEq/L and presence of EKG changes or having serum K+ 6 to 6.4 in the absence of EKG changes. Severe hyperkalemia is defined as either having serum K+ 6 to 6.4 mEq/L and presence of EKG changes or having serum K+ $\geq$6.5 in the presence or absence of EKG changes.[23]

Hyperkalemia can be asymptomatic, or patients can present with occasional nausea, muscle pain, muscle weakness, palpitations, or paresthesia. Moderate–severe hyperkalemia can change the cardiac rhythm leading to asystole. Electrocardiography (ECG) monitoring is essential in moderate–severe hyperkalemia. Typical ECG manifestations include peaked T waves, prolonged PR interval, QRS complex widening, followed by sinewave appearance, ventricular fibrillation, and asystole.[23,25]

Management of hyperkalemia depends on acuity, serum potassium levels, and clinical presentation. Non-pharmacologic interventions include treating the underlying cause of hyperkalemia and limiting potassium intake.[23] **Table 4** includes a summary of treatments for hyperkalemia.

Anemia

Anemia is common in CKD and can significantly impact quality of life.[26] The primary pathogenesis is decreased the production of erythropoietin (EPO), which is necessary for erythropoiesis/red-blood cell formation. Other contributory factors include chronic inflammation, iron deficiency, shortened red-blood cell life span, vitamin deficiencies (folate and B12), and blood loss from frequent laboratories and/or hemodialysis (HD). Anemia is diagnosed in adults when hemoglobin (Hgb) concentration is less than 13.0 g/dL in males and less than 12.0 g/dL in females. Symptoms of anemia include fatigue, dyspnea, and decreased exercise capacity. In addition, anemia can cause cardiovascular complications like left ventricular hypertrophy from the reduction in peripheral vascular resistance and increased cardiac output.

Non-pharmacologic interventions include ensuring appropriate dietary intake of iron, folate, and vitamin B12 and the use of blood transfusions when rapid Hgb increase is needed. Transfusions should be avoided, when possible, to minimize the risk of human leukocyte antigen sensitization (reduces likelihood of transplant), iron overload, and infection transmission.[26]

Iron supplementation

Oral or IV iron is first line for management of iron-deficiency anemia. For patients with CKD, iron supplementation should be initiated when a rise in Hgb is needed, ferritin is less than 500 mcg/L and transferrin saturation is less than 30%.[26] Oral iron should be trialed for 1 to 3 months at 200 mg elemental iron/day in divided doses in patients not on HD. Oral iron is generally not effective in patients on HD due to poor GI absorption and increased blood loss. Adverse effects of oral iron are GI in nature, such as abdominal pain/cramping, nausea, and constipation. Food can reduce adverse events but may reduce absorption. IV iron is recommended for non-dialysis patients who failed oral iron and is the first-line treatment of patients on HD. **Table 5** summarizes the available IV iron formulations. Primary concerns with IV iron include anaphylaxis and free iron reactions.[27] There is a potential risk of worsening bacterial infections; avoidance of IV iron during infection is recommended by KDIGO.[26] However, recent publications suggest this may not be as significant a concern as once thought.[28] Thus, IV iron is generally avoided in severe infection.

Erythropoietin-stimulating agents

Erythropoietin-stimulating agents (ESAs) mimic endogenous EPO and stimulate the bone marrow to produce more red blood cells which can decrease the need for blood transfusions. **Table 6** includes a list of ESAs; biosimilars are not included. Clinical trials of ESAs in patients with CKD who are not on HD indicated that targeting higher Hgb levels resulted in worse cardiovascular outcomes (thromboembolic events, hypertension, and tumor growth). Thus, for patients with CKD-non-dialysis-dependent, ESA therapy is recommended only if Hgb less than 9 g/dL and the benefits outweigh risks.

Table 4
Treatments for hyperkalemia[25,34–36]

	Treatment	Mechanism	Adverse Effect	Clinical Pearls
Acute Management	*Calcium (gluconate or chloride)*	Stabilize the cardiac muscles (*Will not affect potassium levels*)	Hypercalcemia (caution)	• Use only if EKG changes (peaked T waves) present • Onset of action: immediate (1–3 min) • Calcium chloride is not preferred due to risk of skin necrosis in cases of extravasation • Patients with digoxin-induced hyperkalemia should be given calcium at slow infusion over 20–30 min
	Intravenous regular insulin	Shifts potassium intracellularly	*Hypoglycemia*	• Administer with glucose (typically dextrose 50%) if blood glucose is < 250 mg/dL • Onset of action: within 20 min • Insulin effect can last for 4–6 h, and kidney impairment can prolong insulin half-life
	Beta-2-adrenergic agonists (eg, albuterol)	Shifts potassium intracellularly	Cardiovascular (palpitations, tremors, increases in heart rate and anxiety) Bronchospasm	• Dose is 50–100x more than that used in respiratory conditions, leading to side effects • onset of action: within 30 min • Less effective than other methods

(*continued on next page*)

Table 4
(*continued*)

Treatment	Mechanism	Adverse Effect	Clinical Pearls
Sodium bicarbonate	Shifts potassium intracellularly by activating the Na+/K + ATPase, correcting underlying metabolic acidemia	Fluid overload and risk metabolic alkalosis	• Data on its effectiveness and safety are controversial • Reserved for patients with acidemia • Use with caution in patients with CKD and heart failure • Onset of action: hours
Intravenous loop diuretics	Inhibits NKCC2 at thick ascending limb of the loop of Henle, thereby increasing potassium excretion in the distal tubules and collecting ducts	Hypovolemia, metabolic acidosis, AKI	• Unpredictable efficacy in the setting of AKI, progressive stages of CKD and heart failure • Onset of action: ~30 min • Reserve for patients with suspected fluid overload
Kidney replacement therapies	Removes potassium from the body	Hypokalemia, volume depletion	• Caution should be taken to avoid reducing serum potassium too rapidly in patients with cardiac conditions including coronary artery disease or arrhythmias • Highly efficacious in reducing serum potassium • Requires several hours to set up (eg, obtain vascular access) • If dialysis is expected to be delayed, other therapies should be instituted until dialysis is begun

Chronic Management of Hyperkalemia	*Sodium polystyrene sulfonate (Kayexalate)*	Exchanges potassium for sodium in the GI tract, promoting potassium excretion. Also binds magnesium and calcium	• Risk of GI adverse events including intestinal necrosis, constipation, and diarrhea. • Fluid overload in patients sensitive to high sodium intake (eg, heart failure) - Risk for aspiration	• Available as an oral suspension and an enema • Rectal formulation not recommended in acute hyperkalemia • Onset of action variable from hours to days • Space by $\geq$ 3 hours before and after other oral medications (gastroparesis may require 6-h separation) • Avoid concurrent use of sorbitol as it may increase risk of intestinal necrosis
	Patiromer (Veltassa)	Exchanges potassium for calcium ions in the GI tact and also binds magnesium	Diarrhea, constipation, abdominal discomfort, flatulence, hypomagnesemia, hypokalemia	• Available as an oral powder for suspension • Onset of action is about 7 h • Administer other oral medications $\geq$3 h before or after dose
	Sodium: zirconium cyclosilicate (Lokelma)	Exchanges potassium for hydrogen and sodium in the GI tract leading to fecal potassium elimination	Edema, hypokalemia	• Available as an oral powder for suspension • Off label for emergent/ severe hyperkalemia (10 g TID for up to 48 h) • Onset of action in ~1 h • Administer other oral medications $\geq$2 h before or after dose

Table 5
Intravenous irons[26,27]

Iron Agent	Comments
Iron dextran (Infed)	• Highest risk of anaphylaxis reactions compared to other IV iron products • BBW for serious anaphylactic reactions • A test dose is required before the first therapeutic dose • May replete iron deficiency in a single dose
Iron sucrose (Venofer)	• Lower risk of hypersensitivity reactions compared with other IV iron preparations
Ferric carboxymaltose (Injectafer)	• Only indicated for non-dialysis patients with iron deficiency • Hypophosphatemia can occur especially with multiple repeated doses • Allows more iron to be administered at one time than iron sucrose, ferumoxytol, or sodium ferric gluconate.
Sodium ferric gluconate (Ferrlecit)	• Only FDA-approved patients on HD • Higher rates of labile iron compared to other IV iron formulations. Higher risk of free iron reactions like hypotension, flushing headache
Ferumoxytol (Feraheme)	• BBW for anaphylaxis/hypersensitivity reactions

Abbreviations: BBW, black box warning; HD, hemodialysis; ND, non-dialysis.

The current goal range is 9 to 11 g/dL. Patients with uncontrolled hypertension should not receive ESAs due to increased thromboembolic risk. ESAs are ineffective in patients with low iron, vitamin B12, or folate stores. These should also be corrected.

Adjust Medications Based on Kidney Function

Kidney impairment can significantly alter pharmacokinetic and pharmacodynamic responses to medications, threatening their efficacy and leading to safety concerns. Patients with progressive kidney disease often take multiple medications, increasing risk of drug interactions, accumulation of toxic metabolites, and alterations in the overall body hemodynamics.

Pharmacokinetics (PK) includes absorption, distribution, metabolism, and excretion by the body. Pharmacodynamics (PD) describes the effects of a drug/metabolite on the body. **Fig. 2** shows the common alterations to PK and PD for patients with CKD. The renal adjustment of medications requires the use of kidney function estimating equations and clinical decision-making. The Cockcroft–Gault equation for estimating creatinine clearance was used for years to determine PK changes for drugs in patients with varying degrees of kidney dysfunction. More recently, eGFR equations have been used in these PK studies. Additional limitations with the PK studies used for dosing adjustments in manufacturer labeling include:

- Underrepresentation of patients with kidney disease in the efficacy and safety studies
- Nonstandard cutoffs for severity of kidney disease leading to different cutoffs for different medications and no alignment with CKD staging
- Standardization of the SCr assay in 2010. Although this led to consistency in SCr measurements, it created challenges interpreting findings from older estimating equations and studies due to the lack of standardization at that time.

Some drug databases provide additional information, including postmarketing data, to allow the clinician the best information for choosing a dose. In 2021, the

Table 6
Erythropoietin-stimulating agents[26]

Agent (Brand)	Notes	Warnings/Concerns with ESA Therapy
Epoetin alfa (Epogen, Procrit, Retacrit)	• Shortest half-life compared with other ESAs	1. BBW • Increased mortality when targeting Hgb >11 g/dL • Increased risk of hypertension • Increased risk of thromboembolic events including stroke, myocardial infarction, deep venous thrombosis, pulmonary embolism • Shortened survival in patients with cancer and/or increased risk of tumor progression or recurrence 2. ESA hyporesponsivness/ESA resistance • Failure to raise serum Hb after the first month of ESA treatment or requiring 2 increases in ESA doses up to 50% beyond the dose at which Hgb was stable • Investigate causes (eg, poor adherence, iron, folate, and serum vitamin B12) 3. Pure red cell aplasia • A rare condition that occurs as a result of epoetin-induced antibody that neutralizes both exogenous and endogenous EPO • Requirement of blood transfusions
Darbepoetin Alfa (Aranesp)	• Approximately 3-fold longer half-life compared with epoetin alpha	
Methoxy polyethylene glycol-epoetin beta (Mircera)	• Longest half-life compared with other ESA agents	

Abbreviations: subQ, subcutaneous; IV, intravenous; ND, not on dialysis; HD, hemodialysis.

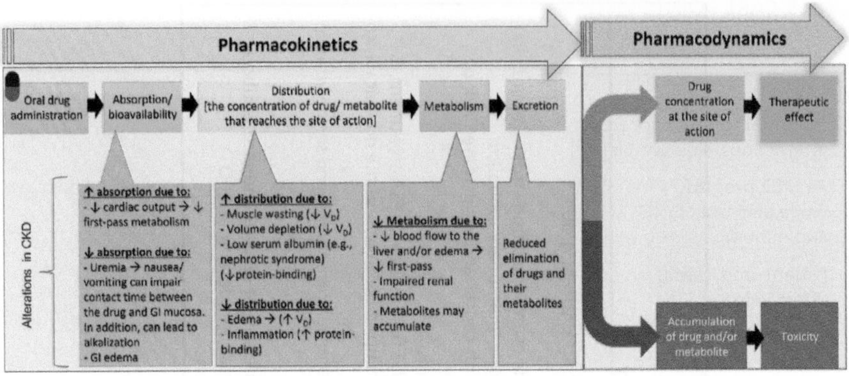

Fig. 2. Common pharmacokinetic and pharmacodynamic alterations in CKD.[32,33] ↑, increase; ↓, decrease; GI, gastrointestinal; V_D, volume of distribution.

National Kidney Foundation and American Society of Nephrology convened a task force to investigate the appropriateness of using black race as a variable in the eGFR equation. They subsequently are recommending the use of the CKD-EPI SCr 2021 equation for CKD staging and increasing the use of cystatin C as a marker of kidney function (https://www.kidney.org/professionals/kdoqi/gfr_calculator).

When choosing a dose for a patient with reduced kidney function, clinicians must use PK study results requiring each dose to be clinically chosen based on the risk of overdosing and underdosing the patient. With these uncertainties, close monitoring for efficacy and toxicity is encouraged.[29,30]

Kidney replacement therapies

Patients who progress to end-stage kidney disease often transition to kidney replacement therapies (KRTs). Available KRT modalities include HD and peritoneal dialysis (PD). Both HD and PD can remove drug from the vascular compartment. Thus, all medications used by patients on KRT must be reviewed for removal during KRT. Sometimes adjustments of frequency and timing of doses can overcome the drug removal. Drug databases contain some information regarding drug removal by various KRT therapies. In general, older drugs are removed to a greater extent by HD than is reported in the prescribing information due to improvements in HD delivery. Frequent assessment of over versus under dosing is required when choosing the best possible dose for a patient followed by close monitoring for safety and efficacy.

SUMMARY

Caring for patients with kidney impairment requires thoughtful regimen design and careful monitoring to ensure positive clinical outcomes. Slowing decline of kidney function using evidenced-based interventions, proactively screening for and treating complications, and making adjustments to the regimen as warranted are strategies for successful management. Engaging a multidisciplinary care team to assist with dietary, social, and medication needs is recommended to manage the complex needs of patients with CKD.

CLINICS CARE POINTS

- People with CKD require complez medication regimens from multiple care providers. It is essiential to check for medication therapy problems at each visit, including dosing, interactions, side effects and adherence concerns.
- As CKD progresses, the clinician should consider interventions to slow progression of CKD while also monitoring for CKD-associated complications, such as anemia, hyperkalemia and mineral and bone disease.
- Patient and caregiver education are integral to ensure medications are used safely and effectively.

DISCLOSURE

L. Salama: Nothing to disclose. S. Sica: Nothing to disclose. K E. Cardone: Advisory board member for AstraZeneca, Otsuka, Vifor; Consultant Wolters Kluwer Kelly, Spouse employed by Fresenius Medical Care; Clinical trial sub-investigator for Merck.

REFERENCES

1. Cardone KE, Manley HJ, Grabe DW, et al. Quantifying home medication regimen changes and quality of life in patients receiving nocturnal home hemodialysis. Hemodial Int 2011;15(2):234–42.
2. Cardone KE, Bacchus S, Assimon MM, et al. Medication-related problems in CKD. Adv Chronic Kidney Dis 2010;17(5):404–12.
3. Manley HJ, Cannella CA, Bailie GR, et al. Medication-related problems in ambulatory hemodialysis patients: a pooled analysis. Am J Kidney Dis 2005;46(4): 669–80.
4. Kidney Disease: Improving Global Outcomes (KDIGO). KDIGO 2012 clinical practice guideline for the evaluation and management of chronic kidney disease. Kidney Int Suppl 2013;3(1):1–150.
5. Ostermann M, Bellomo R, Burdmann EA, et al. Controversies in acute kidney injury: conclusions from a Kidney Disease: improving global outcomes (KDIGO) conference. Kidney Int 2020;98(2):294–309.
6. Kidney Disease: Improving Global Outcomes (KDIGO). KDIGO clinical practice guideline for acute kidney injury. Kidney Int Suppl 2012;2(1).
7. Centers for Disease Control and Prevention. Chronic kidney disease in the United States. Available at: https://www.cdc.gov/kidneydisease/publications-resources/CKD-national-facts.html. Accessed June 14, 2022.
8. KDIGO 2020 clinical practice guideline for diabetes management in chronic kidney disease. Kidney Int 2020;98(4s):S1–115.
9. Bakris GL, Agarwal R, Anker SD, et al. Effect of finerenone on chronic kidney disease outcomes in type 2 diabetes. N Engl J Med 2020;383(23):2219–29.
10. Heerspink HJL, Stefánsson BV, Correa-Rotter R, et al. Dapagliflozin in patients with chronic kidney disease. N Engl J Med 2020;383(15):1436–46.
11. KDIGO. Clinical Practice guideline for the management of blood pressure in chronic kidney disease. Kidney Int 2021;99:S1–87.
12. Cheung AK, Chang TI, Cushman WC, et al. Executive summary of the KDIGO 2021 clinical practice guideline for the management of blood pressure in chronic kidney disease. Kidney Int 2021;99(3):559–69.

13. Weir MR, Bakris GL, Bushinsky DA, et al. Patiromer in patients with kidney disease and hyperkalemia receiving RAAS inhibitors. N Engl J Med 2015;372(3):211–21.
14. Ku E, Lee BJ, Wei J, et al. Hypertension in CKD: core curriculum 2019. Am J Kidney Dis 2019;74(1):120–31.
15. Agarwal R, Sinha AD, Cramer AE, et al. Chlorthalidone for hypertension in advanced chronic kidney disease. N Engl J Med 2021;385(27):2507–19.
16. Chung EY, Ruospo M, Natale P, et al. Aldosterone antagonists in addition to renin angiotensin system antagonists for preventing the progression of chronic kidney disease. Cochrane Database Syst Rev 2020;10(10):CD007004.
17. Pitt B, Filippatos G, Agarwal R, et al. Cardiovascular events with finerenone in kidney disease and type 2 diabetes. N Engl J Med 2021;385(24):2252–63.
18. Agarwal R, Filippatos G, Pitt B, et al. Cardiovascular and kidney outcomes with finerenone in patients with type 2 diabetes and chronic kidney disease: the FIDELITY pooled analysis. Eur Heart J 2022;43(6):474–84.
19. Kidney Disease: Improving Global Outcomes (KDIGO). KDIGO 2017 clinical practice guideline update for the diagnosis, evaluation, prevention, and treatment of chronic kidney disease-mineral and bone disorder (CKD-MBD). Kidney Int Suppl 2017;7(1):1–59.
20. Galassi A, Bellasi A, Ciceri P, et al. Calcifediol to treat secondary hyperparathyroidism in patients with chronic kidney disease. Expert Rev Clin Pharmacol 2017;10(10):1073–84.
21. Quesada-Gomez JM, Bouillon R. Is calcifediol better than cholecalciferol for vitamin D supplementation? Osteoporos Int 2018;29(8):1697–711.
22. Korgaonkar S, Tilea A, Gillespie BW, et al. Serum potassium and outcomes in CKD: insights from the RRI-CKD cohort study. Clin J Am Soc Nephrol 2010;5(5):762–9.
23. Lindner G, Burdmann EA, Clase CM, et al. Acute hyperkalemia in the emergency department: a summary from a Kidney Disease: Improving Global Outcomes conference. Eur J Emerg Med 2020;27(5):329–37.
24. Cupisti A, Kovesdy CP, D'Alessandro C, et al. Dietary approach to recurrent or chronic hyperkalaemia in patients with decreased kidney function. Nutrients 2018;10(3):1–15.
25. Clase CM, Carrero JJ, Ellison DH, et al. Potassium homeostasis and management of dyskalemia in kidney diseases: conclusions from a Kidney Disease: Improving Global Outcomes (KDIGO) Controversies Conference. Kidney Int 2020;97(1):42–61.
26. Kidney Disease: Improving Global Outcomes (KDIGO). KDIGO clinical practice guideline for anemia in chronic kidney disease kidney. Int Suppl 2012;2(4):1–335.
27. Arastu AH, Elstrott BK, Martens KL, et al. Analysis of adverse events and intravenous iron infusion formulations in adults with and without prior infusion reactions. JAMA Netw Open 2022;5(3):e224488.
28. Macdougall IC, Bhandari S, White C, et al. Intravenous iron dosing and infection risk in patients on hemodialysis: a prespecified secondary analysis of the PIVOTAL trial. J Am Soc Nephrol 2020;31(5):1118–27.
29. Cardone KE, Parker WM. Medication management in dialysis: barriers and strategies. Semin Dial 2020;33(6):449–56.
30. Delgado C, Baweja M, Crews DC, et al. A unifying approach for GFR estimation: recommendations of the NKF-ASN task force on reassessing the inclusion of race in diagnosing kidney disease. J Am Soc Nephrol 2021;32(12):2994.

31. Lameire NH, Levin A, Kellum JA, et al. Harmonizing acute and chronic kidney disease definition and classification: report of a Kidney Disease: Improving Global Outcomes (KDIGO) Consensus Conference. Kidney Int 2021;100(3):516–26.
32. Lea-Henry TN, Carland JE, Stocker SL, et al. Clinical pharmacokinetics in kidney disease: fundamental principles. Clin J Am Soc Nephrol 2018;13(7):1085–95.
33. Matzke GR, Aronoff GR, Atkinson AJ, et al. Drug dosing consideration in patients with acute and chronic kidney disease—a clinical update from kidney disease: improving global outcomes (KDIGO). Kidney Int 2011;80(11):1122–37.
34. Sodium polystyrene sulfonate [package insert]. Farmville, NC: CMP Pharma, Inc.; 2021. Available at: https://dailymed.nlm.nih.gov/dailymed/drugInfo.cfm?setid=12d48dcf-07bd-4b06-bd6c-7543f1be8357. Accessed June 23, 2022.
35. Lokelma (sodium zirconium cyclosilicate) [package insert]. Wilmingon, DE: AstraZeneca. 2021. Available at: https://den8dhaj6zs0e.cloudfront.net/50fd68b9-106b-4550-b5d0-12b045f8b184/6de8f71b-d3af-4f76-9600-907c98616be6/6de8f71b-d3af-4f76-9600-907c98616be6_viewable_rendition__v.pdf. Accessed June 23, 2022.
36. Veltassa (patiromer) [package insert]. Redwood City, CA: Vifor Pharma, Inc.; 2021. Available at: https://veltassa.com/themes/custom/veltassa_patient/pdfs/pi.pdf. Accessed June 23, 2022.

What Is Precision Medicine?

Mattie C. Kilpatrick, Pharm.D. Candidate 2023,
Shelton K. Givens, Pharm.D. Candidate 2023,
Courtney S. Watts Alexander, Pharm.D., BCPS, BCOP*

KEYWORDS

- Pharmacogenetics • Pharmacogenomics • Precision medicine
- Personalized medicine

KEY POINTS

- Precision medicine looks to advance health care from a "one-size-fits-all" approach to incorporating genetic, lifestyle, and environmental factors that affect a patient's risk for specific conditions and treatment efficacy and toxicity.
- Pharmacogenomics is a part of precision medicine that assesses the impact of genetic variation on medication response.
- Many drugs, including ones used for conditions related to cardiology, analgesia, mental health, gastroenterology, oncology, immunology, neurology, and infectious diseases, are impacted by pharmacogenomics.
- Precision medicine requires the diverse expertise of multiple health care team members, including prescribers, pharmacists, and genetic counselors, for successful application.

INTRODUCTION

In 2004, the Human Genome Project was declared finished with a nearly complete genome sequence being published. This concluded more than a decade of effort by the United States National Human Genome Research Institute (NHGRI) and the Department of Energy (DOE) in collaboration with the International Human Genome Sequencing Consortium.[1] Nearly a decade later, in January 2015, during President Barack Obama's State of the Union Address, the "Precision Medicine Initiative" was announced with a budget of $215 million to enable further advancement in health care by exploring the impact of variation in individuals' genomic sequences on health.[2] Ultimately, precision medicine seeks to advance health care from a "one-size-fits-all" approach to incorporating genetic, lifestyle, and environmental factors into patient care. These patient-specific factors influence individuals' risk for specific conditions and response to treatment. Pharmacogenomics is a piece of precision medicine that assesses the impact of genetic factors on medication response. This article aimed

Auburn University Harrison College of Pharmacy, Auburn University, 2155 Walker Building, AL 36849, USA
* Corresponding author.
E-mail address: csw0015@auburn.edu

Physician Assist Clin 8 (2023) 371–390
https://doi.org/10.1016/j.cpha.2022.10.013
2405-7991/23/Published by Elsevier Inc.
physicianassistant.theclinics.com

to provide a brief overview of pharmacogenomics with a focus on enzymes and transporters responsible for the action, breakdown, and elimination of common medications. A particular emphasis is placed on specific recommendations provided by either consensus guidelines or the US Food and Drug Administration (FDA) labeling.

Pharmacogenomics Primer

Although the terms pharmacogenomics and pharmacogenetics are often used interchangeably, pharmacogenetics refers to the impact of variation in a single gene. In contrast, pharmacogenomics refers to variations in multiple genes up to the whole genome on medication efficacy or toxicity. To better understand pharmacogenomics, a review of genetic terminology is advised.

The human genome

The human genome is composed of a complete set of genetic materials. The building blocks of DNA are called nucleotides and include adenine, cytosine, guanine, and thymine. Nucleotide sequences form genes that are regions of DNA that provide instructions for creating proteins. Multiple genes are grouped onto chromosomes, and finally, the 23 pairs of chromosomes in each human cell make up the human genome. The first 22 pairs of chromosomes are called autosomes, and the last pair is called sex chromosomes. We use the term allele to describe the sequence at each position on each chromosome, and because we have two copies of each chromosome, we have two alleles at each location.

Through the human genome project, a DNA reference sequence was developed. Although much of DNA is identical between individuals, variation in DNA allows for unique interindividual attributes. The term wild-type refers to the reference allele that is the most common inherited form of the allele. A variant allele indicates an alteration from the wild-type and may lead to a change in the activity of that allele. In pharmacogenomics, star allele nomenclature is used to describe an individual's allelic variation. For example, an individual who inherits a wild-type allele would be said to carry a *1 allele. For each gene, each known variant is assigned a number. These numbers are then categorized based on function. In 2017, the Clinical Pharmacogenetics Implementation Consortium (CPIC) proposed standard terms for characterizing pharmacogenomic allele function. Standardized terms for describing allele function include increased function, normal function, decreased function, no function, unknown function, or uncertain function.[3] Individual genes can also be assigned an activity score; however, the assignment of activity scores is beyond the scope of this review.

To describe an individual's inherited alleles, a genotype is used. A genotype is the pair of alleles an individual carries at a specific location on the DNA. For example, a wild-type, or fully functional genotype would be indicated as *1*1 in star allele nomenclature. A genotype containing two identical alleles is referred to as a homozygous genotype. Conversely, a genotype containing two different alleles is referred to as a heterozygous genotype. Finally, an individual's phenotype is an observable or measurable characteristic resulting from both genetic and environmental influences. Within the field of pharmacogenomics, an individual's genotype is used to provide a predicted phenotype. For details regarding the standardized phenotype terminology used in pharmacogenomics (see **Table 1**).[3]

Standard nomenclature has been defined and used across various genes to maintain consistency. The cytochrome P450 (CYP450) superfamily uses a standard method to name individual members. For example, for the enzyme CYP2D6, "CYP" indicates the superfamily, the number 2 indicates the gene family, the letter D indicates

Table 1
Standardized phenotype nomenclature and descriptions[3]

Gene	Standardized Phenotype Nomenclature	Definition	Implication on a Medication
Drug-metabolizing enzymes (CYP2C9, CYP2C19, CYP2D6, CYP3A5, DPYD, TPMT, UGT1A1)	UM (ultrarapid metabolizer)	Activity increased compared with RM; typically composed of 2 increased function alleles or >2 copies of normal function alleles.	Active drugs may experience increased clearance and reduced effect. Prodrugs may experience increased formation of active metabolites and increased toxicity.
	RM (rapid metabolizer)	Activity increased compared with NM but decreased compared with UM; typically composed of a combination of both normal and increased function alleles.	Active drugs may experience increased clearance and reduced effect. Prodrugs may experience increased formation of active metabolites and increased toxicity.
	NM (normal metabolizer)	Typical functional enzyme activity; typically composed of combinations of normal and/or decreased function alleles.	Typical medication effect.
	IM (intermediate metabolizer)	Activity decreased compared with NM but increased compared with PM; typically composed of combinations of normal, decreased, and/or no function alleles	Active drugs may experience decreased clearance and increased toxicity. Prodrugs may experience decreased formation of active metabolites and reduced effect.
	PM (poor metabolizer)	Little or no enzyme activity; typically composed of combinations of no function or decreased function alleles	Active drugs may experience decreased clearance and increased toxicity. Prodrugs may experience decreased formation of active metabolites and reduced effect.

(*continued on next page*)

Table 1 (continued)

Gene	Standardized Phenotype Nomenclature	Definition	Implication on a Medication
Transporter function (SLCO1B1)	Increased	Increased transporter activity	Increased movement of medication across a membrane; result dependent upon specific medication
	Normal	Typical transporter activity	Typical medication effect.
	Decreased	Decreased transporter activity	Decreased movement of medication across a membrane; result dependent upon specific medication
	Poor	Little or no transporter activity	Little or no movement of medication across a membrane; result dependent upon specific medication
High-risk genotype (HLA)	Positive	High-risk allele detected	Patient inherited 1 (heterozygous) or 2 (homozygous) copies of high-risk allele putting them at increased risk for adverse effect.
	Negative	No high-risk allele detected	Patient did not inherit any high-risk alleles. Standard risk for adverse effect.

the subfamily, and the number 6 indicates the individual gene. Cytochromes are enzymes. Enzymes are proteins that speed up chemical reactions in the body. Another pharmacogenomic target is a transporter. Transporters are proteins embedded in cell membranes that are responsible for the influx and efflux of endogenous and exogenous compounds.[4]

Ultimately, pharmacogenomics is just a "piece of the puzzle." Although pharmacogenomics provides guidance in drug selection, dosing, and monitoring, prescribers must always consider additional patient-specific factors such as renal or hepatic impairment, advanced age, and drug–drug interactions in conjunction with pharmacogenomic data.

Role of Health Care Professionals in Pharmacogenomics

With improved genomic technologies and increased media attention, health care providers will be increasingly presented with requests from patients for genomic testing related to both disease risk and medication response. The direct-to-consumer testing market continues to expand, including options to obtain pharmacogenomic results without health care provider intervention. It is essential that health care providers obtain a general knowledge of pharmacogenomics; however, an understanding of reputable resources is also recommended given the rapidity of change within the science.[5]

Testing

Upon determining that a pharmacogenomic test may be helpful in the selection of pharmacotherapy for a patient, one must make several decisions related to test selection. Any test to be used in the clinical care of a patient should come from a College of American Pathologists (CAP), and Clinical Laboratory Improvement Amendments (CLIA) certified laboratory to ensure testing precision, accuracy, and reliability of results. Types of tests and laboratories can be found using the National Center for Biotechnology Information (NCBI) Genetic Testing Registry (GTR) found at https://www.ncbi.nlm.nih.gov/gtr/.[6] Pharmacogenomic tests can be performed using blood, saliva, or a buccal swab sample. It is rare for institutions to perform pharmacogenomic testing on-site; however, many institutions have preferred vendors. The individual laboratory providing the test can provide specific information related to the processing and stability of the sample and any benefits or limitations to the various specimen types, such as sample stability and incidence of insufficient DNA within the sample.

A single-gene test is typically the least expensive option and determines the patient's genotype and predicted phenotype for a single gene, appropriate for assessing response to an individual drug-gene pair. Multi-gene pharmacogenomic panels are also available. A panel provides a patient's genotype and predicted phenotype for multiple genes with a single specimen. Although a single gene test typically costs less in the short term, the cost of a multi-gene panel approximates the price of two single-gene gene tests and may be more cost-effective over time.

When selecting a pharmacogenomic test, one must critically evaluate the limitations of the panel. Some pertinent questions to ask include:

- What genes are assessed?
- Are these genes clinically relevant and supported by primary literature or evidence-based practice guidelines?
- Are the alleles assessed appropriate for the ethnic ancestry of the target patient population?
- Are any potential incidental findings associated with the genes included on the panel?

Preemptive versus reactive testing

Preemptive pharmacogenomic testing is typically obtained via a multi-gene panel before a patient requires a medication. The goal of preemptive testing is to allow pharmacogenomic information to be available at the point of prescribing, leading to more informed prescribing decisions, improved efficacy, and reduced toxicity. Conversely, reactive testing is performed at the time of prescribing or upon identification of altered response in an individual patient. This can be done as either single-gene testing or via a multi-gene panel. Prescribers should pay particular attention to the testing turnaround time when reactive pharmacogenomic testing is performed to ensure that the patient does not experience harm while waiting for results.

Communication of results

The diverse expertise of the health care team is crucial in implementing precision medicine. Prescribers, pharmacists, and genetic counselors must collaborate to best incorporate pharmacogenomic results into practice.[5,7] The use of pharmacogenomics aims to prevent therapy failure, adverse drug events (ADEs), and medication toxicities, determine appropriate alternative therapies, and identify interacting pharmacologic and non-pharmacological factors. Pharmacists' knowledge of pharmacokinetics and pharmacodynamics places them in the ideal position to lead pharmacogenomic clinical applications to optimize pharmacotherapy and educate both patients and fellow health care team members.[7,8] Playing a different role in the application of precision medicine, genetic counselors use genetic data to interpret risks and possible disease implications and appropriately communicate the significance of results in a patient-centered manner. Overall, precision medicine has the potential to increase patient confidence in their treatment regimen, improve medication adherence, and enhance one's health.[7]

Pharmacogenomics Resources

Given the rapid advancements in pharmacogenomics, health care providers must know where to turn for evidence-based information. Some of the most common resources are described below. Practitioners should use these resources in combination to ensure the most accurate and up-to-date clinical applicability.

The FDA provides the "Table of Pharmacogenomic Biomarkers in Drug Labeling," a database of medications containing pharmacogenomic information in the FDA-approved labeling.[9] Unfortunately, there is no consistent location for this information, nor consistently concrete information describing specific dose adjustments within the labeling. This database assists clinicians in locating pharmacogenomic information efficiently.

Additional databases exist for locating pharmacogenomic information. The Pharmacogenomics Knowledge Base (PharmGKB) is a public database maintained by Stanford University that incorporates data from various sources, including primary, secondary, and tertiary literature. This website is user-friendly with searchable sections including prescribing information, drug label annotations, pharmacokinetic and pharmacodynamic pathways, variant annotations, literature links, and grading of clinical evidence.[10] The Pharmacogene Variation Consortium (PharmVar) was created to catalog variant alleles and provide standardized nomenclature for variants.[11]

The Clinical Pharmacogenomics Implementation Consortium (CPIC) can be consulted for evidence-based clinical practice guidelines. CPIC is an international consortium group based out of the US that guides the use of pharmacogenomic test results in clinical care. CPIC was established with the assumption that pharmacogenomic data would become a standard piece of information available at the point of prescribing, and evidence-based guidelines would be necessary to ensure consistency in the interpretation and utilization of pharmacogenomic information.[12] Additional groups, such as the Dutch Pharmacogenetics Working Group (DPWG) and the Canadian Pharmacogenomics Network for Drug Safety Consortium (CPNDS), also provide consensus guidelines for clinical use. Each of these guidelines can be located via PharmGKB as well. CPIC, PharmGKB, and PharmVar are all supported by National Institutes of Health (NIH) funding.

Application of Pharmacogenomic Principles

Medications used across a multitude of conditions have pharmacogenomic-guided recommendations. This article addresses medications in cardiology, analgesia, mental health, gastroenterology, oncology, immunology, neurology, and infectious diseases. The medications discussed in this article are not an exhaustive list, but the authors aim to provide an overview of current data and strategies for finding new recommendations as the science advances.

Glucose-6-phosphate dehydrogenase

Glucose-6-phosphate dehydrogenase (G6PD) deficiency is an X-linked genetic abnormality and was one of the first described cases in which genetic variation could predict the risk of ADEs for a medication.[10] Although the adverse outcomes associated with

G6PD deficiency were initially discovered following the administration of the medication primaquine in the 1950s, it is Pythagoras who is attributed to describing adverse effects following fava bean ingestion more than 2000 years ago. This non-random hemolytic reaction is now known to be related to a deficiency in the enzyme G6PD. Although individuals carrying deficient G6PD alleles can be found globally, the locations with the highest prevalence include southern Europe, the middle east, southeast Asia, and Africa.[13] Given the large quantity of literature available on this topic, the authors refer to review articles[13,14] devoted to G6PD deficiency for a more in-depth analysis of risk based on both the individual compound and patient-specific genetic variation.[14]

Human Leukocyte Antigen Variation

Variations in the human leukocyte antigen (HLA) have implications for hypersensitivity reactions among many different drug classes. A significant limitation of some medications, including the ones discussed in **Table 2**, is the increased risk of severe cutaneous adverse reactions (SCAR) such as toxic epidermal necrolysis (TEN) and Stevens-Johnson Syndrome (SJS). The risk of SCAR for the below medications is associated with HLA variation. If a variant allele is detected, the implicated medication should be avoided due to the potential for a life-threatening hypersensitivity reaction. Some HLA allelic variations are more prevalent in specific ethnic ancestries, as denoted in **Table 2**. Because of this, testing for HLA variation is recommended in high-risk ancestries before initiating allopurinol, carbamazepine, oxcarbazepine, phenytoin, fosphenytoin, or abacavir.[15–20]

Cardiology Medications

Clopidogrel pharmacogenomics

Clopidogrel is an ideal representation of pharmacogenomics clinical application. Clopidogrel is a prodrug and requires CYP2C19 metabolism for conversion to the pharmacologically active metabolite. An intermediate metabolizer (IM) or poor metabolizer (PM) phenotype for CYP2C19 results in reduced formation of the active metabolite, risking insufficient inhibition of platelet aggregation and increasing the risk for adverse cerebrovascular events. Clopidogrel should be avoided in patients with reduced CYP2C19 function. Alternative antiplatelet therapy, such as prasugrel or ticagrelor, should be used in these patients in the absence of contraindications.[21]

Metoprolol pharmacogenomics

Metoprolol, a cardioselective beta-blocker, is primarily metabolized by CYP2D6. Reduced CYP2D6 function results in increased concentrations of metoprolol, decreasing cardioselectivity, and increasing bradycardia incidence.[22] The DPWG recommends slower titration for reduced CYP2D6 function and dose reductions in IM and PM phenotypes to ensure gradual heart rate reduction and reduced incidence of symptomatic bradycardia. Conversely, increased CYP2D6 function will result in faster inactivation of the drug. The DPWG recommends higher target doses, up to a 2.5-fold increase for individuals experiencing inadequate response. Patients receiving a dose increase should be monitored closely for safety and efficacy. Alternatively, affected patients could be prescribed a beta-blocker not impacted by CYP2D6 variation.[10]

Warfarin pharmacogenomics

The oral anticoagulant warfarin has a narrow therapeutic index and is notorious for not playing well with others. Although direct oral anticoagulant use is increasing, warfarin, a vitamin K antagonist, remains one of the most widely prescribed anticoagulants used for the prevention of thromboembolic diseases. As listed in **Table 3**, there are three enzymes that are currently known to affect warfarin sensitivity: vitamin K epoxide

Table 2
Human leukocyte antigen allelic variation impact on medications[15–20]

HLA Allele	Drug	Therapeutic Use	Associated High-Risk Ancestries	Comments
HLA-B*58:01	Allopurinol	Gout, prevention of tumor lysis syndrome	African, Asian (Thai, Chinese, and Korean), Hawaiian/Pacific Islander	Use contraindicated if HLA-B*58:01 is identified.
HLA-B*15:02	Carbamazepine Oxcarbazepine Phenytoin Fosphenytoin	Antiseizure agent Hydantoin antiseizure agent	Oceanian (Australian continent and Pacific Islands), East/South/Central Asian	Use contraindicated if HLA-B*15:02 identified with no prior use. Cautious re-initiation may be considered if HLA-B*15:02 is identified with prior use >3 mo and no evidence of dermatologic reactions.
HLA-B*57:01	Abacavir	Antiviral for human immunodeficiency virus (HIV)	Screening required for all patients before initiation	Use contraindicated if HLA-B*57:01 is identified.

Table 3
Enzymes affecting warfarin sensitivity[23]

Enzyme	Function	Alleles with Ethnic Considerations
CYP2C9	Major metabolizing enzyme of warfarin	CYP2C9*2 and *3: Implications for non-African ancestry CYP2C9*5, *6, *8, and *11: Implications for African ancestry
CYP4F2	Removal of vitamin K from vitamin K cycle	CYP4F2 *3: Implications in those of European and Asian decent
VKORC1	Warfarin competitively inhibits VKORC1 to reduce synthesis of clotting factors	VKORC1-1639G > A: Implications in Caucasians

reductase complex subunit 1 (VKORC1), CYP2C9, and CYP4F2. Variations in these enzymes can widely alter the necessary therapeutic doses of warfarin for a patient and must be considered when pharmacogenomic-guided warfarin dosing is used.[23]

Ethnic ancestry must be considered when applying pharmacogenomics to warfarin dosing as allele frequencies vary across populations. Some alleles that influence warfarin sensitivity and clearance are more common in specific ethnic groups. The CPIC guidelines describe criteria for allele selection based on self-identified ethnic ancestry; however, patients may not identify with or know of their ethnic ancestry.[24–26] Because pharmacogenomic testing is used across ancestral backgrounds, it is important to ensure that all pertinent alleles are included in the pharmacogenomic panel. If the panel is unable to assess a complete set of alleles, pharmacogenomic-guided dosing should not be used. In these cases, prescribers should initiate therapy with typical starting doses. Resources such as www.warfarindosing.org may be used to determine appropriate warfarin dosing based on patient characteristics and genetic factors.[23]

3-hydroxy-3-methylglutaryl coenzyme-A (HMG-CoA)-reductase inhibitors pharmacogenomics

HMG-CoA-reductase inhibitors, often referred to as "statins," are commonly used to lower cholesterol and reduce cardiovascular disease risk. Statins are prescribed by intensity based on an atherosclerotic cardiovascular disease (ASCVD) risk assessment. ADEs are common with statins, and patients may not tolerate the prescribed intensity due to statin-associated muscle symptoms (SAMS). These symptoms may be caused, in part, by genetic variation in both metabolic enzymes and medication transporters. Solute carrier organic anion transporter family member 1B1 (SLCO1B1) is a gene that encodes organic anion transporter protein 1B1 (OATP1B1), the hepatic transporter responsible for the influx of statins from the blood into the liver for clearance.[27–29] ATP binding cassette subfamily G member 2 (ABCG2) encodes for a protein transporter that functions to move compounds into extracellular space.[28,29] Decreased function of either of these transporters may significantly enhance statin exposure leading to SAMS. A brief overview of modifications based on SLCO1B1 function can be found in **Table 4**; however, the CPIC guidelines should be consulted for a more detailed review.[28]

Pain Medications

Nonsteroidal anti-inflammatory drugs

Nonsteroidal anti-inflammatory drugs (NSAIDs) are commonly associated with gastrointestinal, renal, and cardiovascular ADEs. Although all patients are at risk for ADEs, genetic variation can predict and minimize toxicity. Variations in CYP2C9 are associated with altered NSAID concentrations. Because CYP2C9 phenotype influences

Table 4
Summary of recommendations for statins affected by solute carrier organic anion transporter family member 1B1 function[28]

Statin	SLCO1B1 Decreased Function	SLCO1B1 Poor Function
Atorvastatin	Initiate dosing with ≤ 40 mg; if > 40 mg needed, consider combination therapy.[a]	Initiate dosing with ≤ 20 mg; if > 20 mg needed, consider combination therapy[a] or switching to rosuvastatin.
Lovastatin	Prescribe alternative statin; maximum recommended dose is 20 mg/d.	Prescribe alternative statin.
Pitavastatin	Initiate dosing with ≤ 2 mg; if > 2 mg needed, consider an alternative statin or combination therapy.[a]	Initiate dosing with ≤ 1 mg; if > 1 mg needed, consider an alternative statin or combination therapy.[a]
Pravastatin	Prescribe desired starting dose.	Initiate dosing with ≤ 40 mg; if patient tolerating but requires higher potency, consider increased dose, alternative statin, or combination therapy.[a]
Simvastatin	Prescribe alternative statin; maximum recommended dose is 20 mg/d.	Prescribe an alternative statin.
Rosuvastatin[b]	Prescribe desired starting dose. Increased risk of SAMS with doses > 20 mg. Consult CPIC guideline for recommended adjustments in ABCG2 poor function.	Initiate dosing with ≤ 20 mg; if > 20 mg needed, consider combination therapy.[a] Consult CPIC guideline for recommended adjustments in ABCG2 poor function.
Fluvastatin[c]	Prescribe desired starting dose. Increased risk of SAMS with doses >40 mg. Consult CPIC guideline for recommended adjustments in CYP2C9 IM & PM phenotypes.	Initiate dosing with ≤ 40 mg; if patient tolerating but requires higher potency, consider increased dose, alternative statin, or combination therapy.[a] Avoid use in CYP2C9 IM and PM phenotypes. Consult CPIC guideline for additional information.

[a] Combination therapy: maximally tolerated statin with ezetimibe.
[b] Consider rosuvastatin adjustment for ABCG2 poor function in those with SLCO1B1 increased, normal, decreased, and poor function; see CPIC guidelines for determination of appropriate adjustments.
[c] Consider fluvastatin adjustment for CYP2C9 intermediate and poor metabolizers in those with SLCO1B1 increased, normal, decreased, and poor function; see CPIC guidelines for determination of appropriate adjustments.

systemic concentrations and elimination half-life, recommendations are made based on the respective half-lives of each drug. The longer the half-life of the medication, the greater the risk of toxic effects in patients with reduced CYP2C9 function. With all possible therapies, the lowest effective dose should be used for the shortest duration to minimize ADEs. For patients with reduced CYP2C9 function, alternative therapies such as aspirin, naproxen, ketorolac, or sulindac can be considered.[30,31] A brief overview of modifications for NSAIDs based on CYP2C9 function can be found in **Table 5**.

Table 5
CYP2C9 phenotype effect on nonsteroidal anti-inflammatory drugs[30]

NSAID	CYP2C9 IM	CYP2C9 PM
Ibuprofen[a] Celecoxib[b]	Initiate with the lowest recommended starting dose with cautious titration to clinical efficacy.	Initiate 25% to 50% of the lowest recommended starting dose and with careful titration a maximum of 25% to 50% of the maximum recommended dose.
Meloxicam[c]	Reduction to 50% of the lowest recommended starting dose with careful upward titration no more often than every 7 d.	Selection of an alternative agent is recommended.
Piroxicam	Alternative therapy required.	

[a] Dose adjustments should not occur more than every 5 d.
[b] Dose adjustments should not occur more than every 8 d.
[c] Dose adjustments should not occur more than every 7 d.

Opioids

Opioids are known for their use in treating both chronic and acute pain. Interindividual differences in efficacy and ADEs can be, in part, attributed to variations in CYP2D6 activity. Codeine and tramadol are prodrugs that are converted by CYP2D6 into metabolites with increased activity. Because of this, a CYP2D6 UM phenotype results in supratherapeutic concentrations and increased risk for toxicities, for which alternative therapy is recommended. CYP2D6 NMs or IMs do not require dose adjustments, but those with an IM phenotype should be monitored for suboptimal response. Codeine and tramadol should be avoided in those with a CYP2D6 PM phenotype due subtherapeutic concentrations and risk of therapeutic failure.[31]

Mental Health Medications

Selective serotonin reuptake inhibitors

Selective serotonin reuptake inhibitors (SSRIs) are commonly prescribed for many psychiatric conditions; however, due to interindividual variability, discontinuation rates have been reported as high as 70%.[32] In fact, approximately 50% of patients with major depressive disorder experience therapeutic failure after adequate treatment with a first-line SSRI. As patient response to SSRIs can only be assessed after several weeks of continuous therapy, pharmacogenomic-guided medication selection has the potential to lead to improved efficacy and reduced ADEs.[33]

Table 6 provides phenotype-specific dosing recommendations for SSRIs. Generally, a UM phenotype will result in reduced drug concentrations, increasing the probability of therapeutic failure. A PM phenotype will produce elevated drug concentrations, increasing the risk of ADEs. For the SSRIs metabolized by CYP2C19, QTc prolongation is a significant concern. An alternative SSRI metabolized through a different pathway is typically preferred for both UM and PM phenotypes.

Serotonin and norepinephrine reuptake inhibitors

Venlafaxine is a serotonin and norepinephrine reuptake inhibitor (SNRI) that requires adjustment in individuals with a CYP2D6 UM, IM, or PM phenotype. An IM or PM phenotype increases the risk for ADEs, and conservative dosing with close monitoring or an alternative agent may be preferred. A CYP2D6 UM phenotype may require dose titration of up to 150% of the usual dose or an alternative medication.[33]

Table 6
Pharmacogenomic recommendations for selective serotonin reuptake inhibitors[33,34]

Drug	Enzyme	UM Phenotype	PM Phenotype
Citalopram	CYP2C19	Avoid use	If used, maximum dose of 20 mg/d
Escitalopram	CYP2C19	Avoid use	Consider initiation with 50% of standard dose with cautious up titration
Sertraline	CYP2C19	Avoid use	Consider initiation with 50% of standard dose with cautious up titration
Paroxetine	CYP2D6	Consider alternative SSRI.	Consider alternative SSRI.
Fluvoxamine	CYP2D6	Consider alternative SSRI.	Consider alternative SSRI.
Vortioxetine	CYP2D6	No recommendation available.	Maximum dose of 10 mg/d.

Tricyclic antidepressants

Tricyclic antidepressants (TCAs) are mixed serotonin and norepinephrine reuptake inhibitors historically used in major depressive disorder, obsessive-compulsive disorder, and neuropathic pain; however, use has declined due to undesirable ADEs, which may be mitigated by pharmacogenomic-guided individualization. The TCAs can be separated into two groups. The tertiary amines include amitriptyline, imipramine, clomipramine, trimipramine, and doxepin, and are metabolized by CYP2C19 and CYP2D6. The secondary amines include nortriptyline, desipramine, and protriptyline which are only metabolized by CYP2D6. Most pharmacogenomic studies have concentrated on amitriptyline and nortriptyline, which is reflected in current guidelines. However, because other TCAs have comparable pharmacokinetic properties, results and subsequent recommended dose adjustments are similar across the class and are described in **Table 7**.[35] Unfortunately, a paucity of data exists regarding TCA individualization in those with combinations of CYP2D6 and CYP2C19 metabolic variations. Therefore, it is advisable to use therapeutic drug level monitoring (TDM) or consider an alternative medication class.[36]

Antipsychotics

Antipsychotic medications are used for various indications, including augmentation with antidepressants in mood and anxiety disorders, bipolar disorder, schizophrenia,

Table 7
Pharmacogenomic considerations for tricyclic antidepressants[36]

	CYP2D6	CYP2C19
UM phenotype	Alternative agents should be considered due to the risk of treatment failure. If TCA is required, use TDM to guide adjustments.	Alternative agents should be considered due to the risk of treatment failure and ADEs. If TCA is required, use TDM to guide adjustments.
RM phenotype	No specific recommendations.	
IM phenotype	Alternative agents are preferred; reduce dose by 25% if used.	No specific recommendations.
PM phenotype	Alternative agents are preferred; reduce dose by 50% if used.	Alternative agents are preferred; reduce dose by 50% if used.

and an autism spectrum disorder. The antipsychotics with pharmacogenomic considerations, also found in **Table 8**, include first-generation (typical) antipsychotics pimozide and thioridazine and the second-generation (atypical) antipsychotics aripiprazole, brexpiprazole, and iloperidone. These medications are primarily metabolized to inactive metabolites by CYP2D6. In addition to desirable effects, antipsychotics are known to cause side effects related to off-target antagonism, and CYP2D6 phenotypes should be considered when choosing an antipsychotic medication.

Gastrointestinal Medications

Antiemetics

Ondansetron is an antiemetic used in the prevention of nausea and vomiting. CYP2D6 is primarily responsible for ondansetron metabolism to inactive metabolites, and a CYP2D6 UM phenotype results in decreased antiemetic effect. Therefore, those with a CYP2D6 UM phenotype should use an alternative antiemetic. There are no required adjustments for NMs, IMs, or PMs of CYP2D6.[42]

Proton-pump inhibitors

Proton-pump inhibitors (PPIs) are extensively used for acid suppression in several gastrointestinal disorders. Most PPIs, including omeprazole, lansoprazole, pantoprazole, and dexlansoprazole, are metabolized to inactive metabolites by CYP2C19.[43] Individuals with a CYP2C19 UM phenotype require increased doses of up to 100% for therapeutic efficacy. Both CYP2C19 RM and NM phenotypes have been associated with increased risk for therapeutic failure and may require upward dose titration. Conversely, those with a CYP2C19 IM or PM phenotype should receive standard dosing initially with downward dose titration to avoid possible ADEs.[44]

Oncology and Immunosuppressant Medications

Uridine diphosphate glucuronosyltransferase 1 family, polypeptide A1 (UGT1A1) pharmacogenomics

UGT1A1 is an enzyme responsible for glucuronidation allowing for enterohepatic recycling and elimination. Reduced UGT1A1 activity leads to reduced clearance

Table 8
Recommendations for use of antipsychotics in CYP2D6 phenotypes[10,37–41]

Drug	Dosing Recommendations
Pimozide[a]	IM phenotype: Use no more than 80% of the standard maximum dose • 12 y and older: 16 mg/d • Children under 12: 0.08 mg/kg per day (maximum 3 mg/d) PM phenotype: Use no more than 50% of the standard maximum dose. Titrate at intervals of at least 14 d • 12 y and older: 10 mg/d • Children under 12: 0.05 mg/kg per day (maximum 2 mg/d)
Thioridazine	PM phenotype: Use is contraindicated due to increased risk of QTc prolongation and torsades de pointes
Aripiprazole	PM phenotype: Use no more than 50% of usual dose for immediate-release formulation (10 mg/d); maximum 300 mg of extended-release (monthly) injectable formulation
Brexpiprazole	PM phenotype: Use no more than 50% of usual dose
Iloperidone	PM phenotype: Reduce dose by 50%.

[a] Requires genotyping for doses greater than 0.05 mg/kg per day in children or 4 mg/d in adults.

resulting in an increased risk of dose-dependent toxicities of drugs metabolized by UGT1A1.[45]

Belinostat, a histone deacetylase inhibitor, is used to treat certain lymphomas. Patients with homozygous deficient UGT1A1 activity require a reduced starting dose to decrease the risk of dose-limiting toxicities (DLTs).[46] Irinotecan is a topoisomerase inhibitor commonly used in colorectal and pancreatic cancers. UGT1A1 mediates the glucuronidation of the active metabolite, SN-38, to its inactive form. Those with homozygous deficient UGT1A1 activity are at increased risk for neutropenia and should have a reduced starting dose that is dependent on the irinotecan product, indication, and patient-specific treatment tolerance.[47,48] Finally, the tyrosine kinase inhibitor nilotinib is indicated for the treatment of certain leukemias and inhibits UGT1A1. Patients with homozygous deficient UGT1A1 activity are at increased risk for hyperbilirubinemia.[49]

Antimetabolite agents

Both 5-fluorouracil (5-FU) and capecitabine (5-FU prodrug) are pyrimidine antimetabolites used in several malignancies. The rate-limiting step of 5-FU breakdown is the enzyme dihydropyrimidine dehydrogenase (DPD), encoded by the gene DPYD.[50] Decreased DPD activity leads to diminished clearance, a longer half-life, and extensive toxicity.[51] A dose reduction is recommended if a DPYD IM phenotype is identified.[50] Decreased DPD activity leads to diminished clearance, a longer half-life, and extensive toxicity.[51] Fluoropyrimidine antimetabolites should be avoided in those with a PM phenotype due to the increased risk of severe or fatal ADEs.[50]

Thiopurine antimetabolites mercaptopurine, thioguanine, and azathioprine are commonly used in pediatric malignancies or autoimmune conditions. These agents are metabolized by thiopurine methyltransferase (TPMT) and nucleoside diphosphate-linked moiety X-type motif 15 (NUDT15). Reduced TPMT or NUDT15 activity leads to increased risk for ADEs such as myelosuppression and hepatotoxicity.[52] **Table 9** provides general recommendations for thiopurine drugs; however, the CPIC guidelines should be referenced for additional specific information.

Tamoxifen pharmacogenomics

Tamoxifen is an antagonist at estrogen receptors and is used for the treatment of hormone-positive breast cancer. Tamoxifen is a prodrug requiring metabolism by CYP2D6 and CYP3A4/5 to form the active metabolite endoxifen. CYP2D6 deficiency results in reduced endoxifen concentrations, reducing efficacy and increasing risk of relapse or disease progression. Alternative therapy with a class of medications called aromatase inhibitors (combined with ovarian suppression in premenopausal women) should be considered for those with an IM or PM phenotype.[53]

Tacrolimus

Tacrolimus is a commonly used, narrow therapeutic index immunosuppressant indicated for the prevention of transplanted organ rejection. Tacrolimus is predominantly metabolized by CYP3A4 and CYP3A5. CYP3A5 phenotypes are classified as expressers (NM or IM phenotype) or nonexpressers (PM phenotype).[54] CYP3A5 is ethnically linked, with a higher prevalence of variant expression in African American, Southeast Asian, Pacific Islander, and Southwestern American Indian patients.[55] CYP3A5 expressers are at risk for reduced tacrolimus concentrations due to enhanced metabolism. If CYP3A5 genotype is available, CYP3A5 expressers should receive elevated initial doses.[54]

Table 9
Summary of thiopurine drugs[52]

Thiopurine Drug (Utilization)	Dosing Recommendations Based on Pharmacogenomic Genotype			
		TPMT NM	TPMT IM	TPMT PM
Mercaptopurine (malignancy; acute lymphoblastic leukemia)	NUDT15 NM	Standard dosing	Initiate at 30% to 80% of normal dose	Malignant conditions: Initiate 10% of dose and administer thrice weekly Nonmalignant conditions: Consider alternative agent
	NUDT15 IM	Initiate at 30% to 80% of normal dose		
	NUDT15 PM	Malignant conditions: initiate at 10 mg/m^2/d Nonmalignant conditions: consider alternative agent	Malignant conditions: initiate at 10 mg/m^2/d Nonmalignant conditions: consider alternative agent	
Thioguanine (malignancy; acute myeloid leukemia, acute lymphoblastic leukemia)	NUDT15 NM	Standard dosing	Initiate at 50% to 80% of normal dose	
	NUDT15 IM	Initiate at 50% to 80% of normal dose		
	NUDT15 PM	Initiate at 25% of normal dose		
Azathioprine (immunosuppression in autoimmune and rheumatological conditions)	NUDT15 NM	Standard dosing	Initiate at 30% to 80% of normal dose	
	NUDT15 IM	Initiate at 30% to 80% of normal dose		
	NUDT15 PM	Malignant conditions: Initiate 10% of dose daily Nonmalignant conditions: Consider alternative agent		

Neurology Medications

Antiepileptics

Phenytoin and fosphenytoin have been discussed as medications impacted by HLA-B*15:02 allelic variation but are also impacted by CYP2C9 variation. For individuals with a CYP2C9 PM or IM phenotype, reduced doses may be required. Although the dose may be individualized based on patient-specific pharmacogenomic results, TDM is also recommended.[19]

Clobazam is a benzodiazepine anti-seizure agent metabolized by CYP2C19. For patients known to have a CYP2C19 PM phenotype, an initial maximum dose of 5 mg/d with cautious titration is recommended. As this drug is indicated for use in pediatric patients, weight should be considered in selection of appropriate dose and upward titration.[56]

Infectious Disease Medications

Antiviral medications

Atazanavir, an antiviral used in the treatment of human immunodeficiency virus (HIV), prevents glucuronidation of bilirubin by UGT1A1. Increases in bilirubin are common in individuals treated with atazanavir; however, this is not typically an indication of true injury to the liver. Unfortunately, when atazanavir is used in a patient with a UGT1A1 PM phenotype, a significantly increased risk of visually apparent jaundice occurs, increasing risk of discontinuation. As medication adherence is essential in HIV treatment, identification of a UGT1A1 PM phenotype should result in a concern for hyperbilirubinemia, jaundice, and subsequent reduced compliance.[57]

Antifungal medications

Voriconazole is an antifungal agent used in severe, invasive fungal infections such as aspergillosis, candidiasis, scedosporiosis, and fusariosis. The major pathway of metabolism of voriconazole is through the enzyme CYP2C19. Because alterations in metabolism may affect therapeutic efficacy, the CYP2C19 phenotype should be considered when choosing antifungal therapy. For adults with CYP2C19 UM and RM phenotypes, an alternative agent such as posaconazole, isavuconazole, or liposomal amphotericin B should be used. Individuals with a CYP2C19 PM phenotype will experience higher trough concentrations. To reduce toxicity, the use of an alternative agent, as listed above, is recommended; however, voriconazole may be used at a lower dose with TDM and close monitoring for ADEs such as hepatotoxicity, visual disturbances, and hallucinations.[58]

SUMMARY

Precision medicine encompasses a variety of fields, including precision oncology and immunotherapy, pharmacogenomics, and identification and diagnosis of rare diseases. As both drug therapy and genomic testing advance, reduced costs will likely increase accessibility leading to increased focus on interindividual genomic variation in both clinical practice and clinical trial design and implementation. As such, although pharmacogenomics historically has been limited in scope, increased accessibility and focus are likely to increase the number of drug-gene pairs that can be used to individualize therapy, increasing efficacy, and reducing toxicity. Given the magnitude of data and velocity of discovery, interdisciplinary collaboration is essential to incorporate principles of precision medicine into patient care consistently. As precision medicine advances, health care providers practicing within pharmacogenomics will be critical for shifting the model from reactive to preemptive testing and incorporation into initial pharmacotherapeutic decision-making.

CLINICS CARE POINTS

- As further pharmacogenomic research is conducted, recommendations for specific drug-gene pairs may change. It is imperative to be familiar with up-to-date, evidence-based resources, such CPIC Guidelines or PharmGKB, when making recommendations.
- Use of direct-to-consumer testing increases accessibility to genomic results but may not be suitable for utilization in clinical care. When choosing a pharmacogenomic test, consideration should be given to panels that include genes with evidence-based practice guidelines, that are appropriate for a specific patient's ethnic ancestry, and that come from a laboratory that is CLIA and CAP certified.

DISCLOSURE

The authors have no conflicts to disclose.

REFERENCES

1. National Human Genome Research Institute. Talking Glossary of Genetic Terms. Available at. https://www.genome.gov/genetics-glossary. Accessed April 21, 2022.
2. White House The. President Barack Obama. Available at: https://obamawhitehouse.archives.gov/precision-medicine. Accessed April 12, 2022.
3. Caudle KE, Dunnenberger HM, Freimuth RR, et al. Standardizing terms for clinical pharmacogenetic test results: consensus terms from the Clinical Pharmacogenetics Implementation Consortium (CPIC). Genet Med 2017;19(2):215–23.
4. National Cancer Institute. NCI Dictionary of Genetics Terms. Available at. https://www.cancer.gov/publications/dictionaries/genetics-dictionary. Accessed April 21, 2022.
5. Gammal RS, Smith DM, Wiisanen KW, et al. The pharmacist's responsibility to ensure appropriate use of direct-to-consumer genetic testing. J Am Coll Clin Pharm 2021;4(5):652–8.
6. National Library of Medicine (US). National Center for Biotechnology Information. GTR: Genetic Testing Registry. Available at: https://www.ncbi.nlm.nih.gov/gtr/. Accessed June 9, 2022.
7. Chart NA, Kisor DF, Farrell CL. Defining the role of pharmacists in medication-related genetic counseling. Per Med 2021;18(5):509–22.
8. Tillman EM, Beavers CJ, Afanasjeva J, et al. Current and future state of clinical pharmacist-led precision medicine initiatives. J Am Coll Clin Pharm 2021;4(6):754–64.
9. U.S. Food & Drug Administration. Table of Pharmacogenomic Biomarkers in Drug Labeling. Available at. https://www.fda.gov/drugs/science-and-research-drugs/table-pharmacogenomic-biomarkers-drug-labeling. Accessed April 21, 2022.
10. Whirl-Carrillo M, Huddart R, Gong L, et al. An Evidence-Based Framework for Evaluating Pharmacogenomics Knowledge for Personalized Medicine. Clin Pharmacol Ther 2021;110(3):563–72.
11. Pharmacogene PharmVar. Variation Consortium. The PharmVar Consortium. Available at. https://www.pharmvar.org/about. Accessed April 21, 2022.

12. Relling MV, Klein TE. CPIC: Clinical Pharmacogenetics Implementation Consortium of the Pharmacogenomics Research Network. Clin Pharmacol Ther 2011;89(3):464–7.
13. Luzzatto L, Arese P. Favism and glucose-6-phosphate dehydrogenase deficiency. N Engl J Med 2018;378(1):60–71.
14. Luzzatto L, Ally M, Notaro R. Glucose-6-phosphate dehydrogenase deficiency. Blood 2020;136(11):1225–40.
15. Keller SF, Lu N, Blumenthal KG, et al. Racial/ethnic variation and risk factors for allopurinol-associated severe cutaneous adverse reactions: a cohort study. Ann Rheum Dis 2018;77(8):1187–93.
16. Hershfield MS, Callaghan JT, Tassaneeyakul W, et al. Clinical Pharmacogenetics Implementation Consortium guidelines for human leukocyte antigen-B genotype and allopurinol dosing. Clin Pharmacol Ther 2013;93(2):153–8.
17. Saito Y, Stamp LK, Caudle KE, et al. Clinical Pharmacogenetics Implementation Consortium (CPIC) guidelines for human leukocyte antigen B (HLA-B) genotype and allopurinol dosing: 2015 update. Clin Pharmacol Ther 2016;99(1):36–7.
18. Phillips EJ, Sukasem C, Whirl-Carrillo M, et al. Clinical Pharmacogenetics Implementation Consortium Guideline for HLA Genotype and Use of Carbamazepine and Oxcarbazepine: 2017 Update. Clin Pharmacol Ther 2018;103(4):574–81.
19. Karnes JH, Rettie AE, Somogyi AA, et al. Clinical Pharmacogenetics Implementation Consortium (CPIC) Guideline for CYP2C9 and HLA-B Genotypes and Phenytoin Dosing: 2020 Update. Clin Pharmacol Ther 2021;109(2):302–9.
20. Martin MA, Klein TE, Dong BJ, et al. Clinical pharmacogenetics implementation consortium guidelines for HLA-B genotype and abacavir dosing. Clin Pharmacol Ther 2012;91(4):734–8.
21. Lee CR, Luzum JA, Sangkuhl K, et al. Clinical Pharmacogenetics Implementation Consortium Guideline for CYP2C19 Genotype and Clopidogrel Therapy: 2022 Update. Clin Pharmacol Ther 2022. https://doi.org/10.1002/cpt.2526.
22. Toprol-XL (metoprolol succinate) tablet, extended-release for oral use [package insert]. Wilmington, DE: AstraZeneca. Available at: https://www.accessdata.fda.gov/drugsatfda_docs/label/2009/019962s038lbl.pdf. Accessed June 22, 2022.
23. Johnson JA, Caudle KE, Gong L, et al. Clinical Pharmacogenetics Implementation Consortium (CPIC) Guideline for Pharmacogenetics-Guided Warfarin Dosing: 2017 Update. Clin Pharmacol Ther 2017;102(3):397–404.
24. Drozda K, Wong S, Patel SR, et al. Poor warfarin dose prediction with pharmacogenetic algorithms that exclude genotypes important for African Americans. Pharmacogenet Genomics 2015;25(2):73–81.
25. Perera MA, Cavallari LH, Limdi NA, et al. Genetic variants associated with warfarin dose in African-American individuals: a genome-wide association study. Lancet 2013;382(9894):790–6.
26. Pratt VM, Cavallari LH, Del Tredici AL, et al. Recommendations for Clinical Warfarin Genotyping Allele Selection: A Report of the Association for Molecular Pathology and the College of American Pathologists. J Mol Diagn 2020;22(7):847–59.
27. Oshiro C, Mangravite L, Klein T, et al. PharmGKB very important pharmacogene: SLCO1B1. Pharmacogenet Genomics 2010;20(3):211–6.
28. Cooper-DeHoff RM, Niemi M, Ramsey LB, et al. The Clinical Pharmacogenetics Implementation Consortium Guideline for SLCO1B1, ABCG2, and CYP2C9 genotypes and Statin-Associated Musculoskeletal Symptoms. Clin Pharmacol Ther 2022;111(5):1007–21.

29. Fohner AE, Brackman DJ, Giacomini KM, et al. PharmGKB summary: very important pharmacogene information for ABCG2. Pharmacogenet Genomics 2017; 27(11):420–7.
30. Theken KN, Lee CR, Gong L, et al. Clinical Pharmacogenetics Implementation Consortium Guideline (CPIC) for CYP2C9 and Nonsteroidal Anti-Inflammatory Drugs. Clin Pharmacol Ther 2020;108(2):191–200.
31. Crews KR, Monte AA, Huddart R, et al. Clinical Pharmacogenetics Implementation Consortium Guideline for CYP2D6, OPRM1, and COMT Genotypes and Select Opioid Therapy. Clin Pharmacol Ther 2021;110(4):888–96.
32. Mullins CD, Shaya FT, Meng F, et al. Persistence, switching, and discontinuation rates among patients receiving sertraline, paroxetine, and citalopram. Pharmacotherapy 2005;25(5):660–7.
33. Hicks JK, Bishop JR, Sangkuhl K, et al. Clinical Pharmacogenetics Implementation Consortium (CPIC) Guideline for CYP2D6 and CYP2C19 Genotypes and Dosing of Selective Serotonin Reuptake Inhibitors. Clin Pharmacol Ther 2015; 98(2):127–34.
34. Trintellix (vortioxetine) tablets [package insert]. Lexington, MA: Takeda Pharmaceuticals America, Inc.. Available at: https://general.takedapharm.com/TRINTELLIXPI. Accessed June 22, 2022.
35. Stingl JC, Brockmöller J, Viviani R. Genetic variability of drug-metabolizing enzymes: the dual impact on psychiatric therapy and regulation of brain function. Mol Psychiatry 2013;18(3):273–87.
36. Hicks JK, Sangkuhl K, Swen JJ, et al. Clinical pharmacogenetics implementation consortium guideline (CPIC) for CYP2D6 and CYP2C19 genotypes and dosing of tricyclic antidepressants: 2016 update. Clin Pharmacol Ther 2017;102(1):37–44.
37. Orap (pimozide) tablet [package insert]. Sellersville, PA: Teva Pharmaceuticals USA. Available at: https://www.accessdata.fda.gov/drugsatfda_docs/label/2009/017473s041lbl.pdf. Accessed on June 22, 2022.
38. Thioridazine hydrochloride tablet [package insert]. Rockford, IL: Mylan Pharmaceuticals Inc. Available at: https://dailymed.nlm.nih.gov/dailymed/drugInfo.cfm?setid=52fea941-0b47-41c1-b00d-f88150e8ab93. Accessed on June 22, 2022.
39. Abilify (aripiprazole) [package insert]. Rockville, MD: Otsuka America Pharmaceutical, Inc. Available at: https://www.otsuka-us.com/sites/g/files/qhldwo5261/files/media/static/Abilify-M-PI.pdf. Accessed on June 22, 2022.
40. Rexulti (brexpiprazole) [package insert]. Rockville, MD: Otsuka America Pharmaceutical, Inc. Available at: https://otsuka-us.com/sites/g/files/qhldwo5261/files/media/static/Rexulti-PI.pdf. Accessed June 22, 2022.
41. Fanapt (iloperidone) tablet [package insert]. Washington, D.C: Vanda Pharmaceuticals Inc. Available at: https://fanaptpro.com/wp-content/uploads/2016/02/Fanapt-Prescribing-Information.pdf. Accessed June 22, 2022.
42. Bell GC, Caudle KE, Whirl-Carrillo M, et al. Clinical Pharmacogenetics Implementation Consortium (CPIC) guideline for CYP2D6 genotype and use of ondansetron and tropisetron. Clin Pharmacol Ther 2017;102(2):213–8.
43. El Rouby N, Lima JJ, Johnson JA. Proton pump inhibitors: from CYP2C19 pharmacogenetics to precision medicine. Expert Opin Drug Metab Toxicol 2018; 14(4):447–60.
44. Lima JJ, Thomas CD, Barbarino J, et al. Clinical Pharmacogenetics Implementation Consortium (CPIC) Guideline for CYP2C19 and Proton Pump Inhibitor Dosing. Clin Pharmacol Ther 2021;109(6):1417–23.

45. Barbarino JM, Haidar CE, Klein TE, et al. PharmGKB summary: very important pharmacogene information for UGT1A1. Pharmacogenet Genomics 2014;24(3): 177–83.
46. Beleodaq (belinostat) for injection, for intravenous use [package insert]. Irvine, CA: Spectrum Pharmaceuticals, Inc. Available at: https://www.accessdata.fda.gov/drugsatfda_docs/label/2014/206256lbl.pdf/. Accessed June 22, 2022.
47. Camptosar (irinotecan) injection, intravenous infusion [package insert]. New York, New York: Pharmacia & Upjohn Co. Division of Pfizer Inc. Available at: https://www.accessdata.fda.gov/drugsatfda_docs/label/2014/020571s048lbl.pdf. Accessed June 22, 2022.
48. Onivyde (irinotecan liposome injection), for intravenous use [package insert]. Basking Ridge, NJ: Ispen Biopharmaceuticals, Inc. Available at: https://www.ipsen.com/websites/Ipsen_Online/wp-content/uploads/sites/9/2019/01/21083350/ONIVYDE_USPI.pdf. Accessed June 22, 2022.
49. Tasigna (nilotinib) capsules, for oral use [package insert]. East Hanover, NJ: Novartis Pharmaceuticals Corporation. Available at: https://www.accessdata.fda.gov/drugsatfda_docs/label/2007/022068lbl.pdf. Accessed June 22, 2022.
50. Amstutz U, Henricks LM, Offer SM, et al. Clinical Pharmacogenetics Implementation Consortium (CPIC) Guideline for Dihydropyrimidine Dehydrogenase Genotype and Fluoropyrimidine Dosing: 2017 Update. Clin Pharmacol Ther 2018; 103(2):210–6.
51. Boisdron-Celle M, Remaud G, Traore S, et al. 5-Fluorouracil-related severe toxicity: A comparison of different methods for the pretherapeutic detection of dihydropyrimidine dehydrogenase deficiency. Cancer Lett 2007;249(2):271–82.
52. Relling MV, Schwab M, Whirl-Carrillo M, et al. Clinical Pharmacogenetics Implementation Consortium Guideline for Thiopurine Dosing Based on TPMT and NUDT15 Genotypes: 2018 Update. Clin Pharmacol Ther 2019;105(5):1095–105.
53. Goetz MP, Sangkuhl K, Guchelaar HJ, et al. Clinical Pharmacogenetics Implementation Consortium (CPIC) Guideline for CYP2D6 and Tamoxifen Therapy. Clin Pharmacol Ther 2018;103(5):770–7.
54. Birdwell KA, Decker B, Barbarino JM, et al. Clinical Pharmacogenetics Implementation Consortium (CPIC) Guidelines for CYP3A5 Genotype and Tacrolimus Dosing. Clin Pharmacol Ther 2015;98(1):19–24.
55. Kuehl P, Zhang J, Lin Y, et al. Sequence diversity in CYP3A promoters and characterization of the genetic basis of polymorphic CYP3A5 expression. Nat Genet 2001;27(4):383–91.
56. Onfi (clobazam) [package insert]. Winchester, KY: Catalent Pharma Solutions, LLC. Available at: https://www.accessdata.fda.gov/drugsatfda_docs/label/2016/203993s005lbl.pdf. Accessed June 22, 2022.
57. Gammal RS, Court MH, Haidar CE, et al. Clinical Pharmacogenetics Implementation Consortium (CPIC) Guideline for UGT1A1 and Atazanavir Prescribing. Clin Pharmacol Ther 2016;99(4):363–9.
58. Moriyama B, Obeng AO, Barbarino J, et al. Clinical Pharmacogenetics Implementation Consortium (CPIC) Guidelines for CYP2C19 and Voriconazole Therapy. Clin Pharmacol Ther 2017;102(1):45–51.

Explaining Insurance and the Medication Pipeline

Lena McDowell, PharmD[a,*], Mafe Zmajevac, PharmD[b]

KEYWORDS

• Medication • Investigational new drug • New drug application • Drug coverage
• Insurance • Pharmacy benefit manager • Social determinants of health
• Patient assistance

KEY POINTS

- The United States Food and Drug Administration oversees the approval of new drugs with a 5-step systematic process to ensure they are safe and effective for consumers.
- Pharmaceutical compounds and dietary products, such as herbal supplements and vitamins, follow different approval regulations.
- Insurance and prescription drug coverage is available through a variety of avenues, including government-funded programs such as Medicare and Medicaid as well as employer-sponsored and individual plans through private insurance companies.
- Medication affordability is a widespread issue, affecting millions of Americans each day.
- Social determinants of health contribute to health disparities, including lack of medication access.

INTRODUCTION

Approximately half of Americans indicated they have used at least one prescription drug within the preceding month.[1] Twenty percent of all new prescriptions are never filled, and of the prescriptions that are dispensed to patients, only half are taken correctly, resulting in poor patient outcomes.[2] One of the contributing factors to medication nonadherence is patients' lack of access to medications. Healthy People 2030 recognizes financial barriers and lack of insurance coverage as reasons people are unable to access the medications they need. The organization has set target goals to increase the proportion of people in the United States (US) with health and prescription drug insurance and reduce the proportion of people who cannot obtain prescription medications when they need them.[3–5] Health-care providers are positioned to identify social determinants of health contributing to medication access issues and assist

[a] Auburn University Harrison College of Pharmacy, Auburn University, 2137 Walker Building, Auburn, AL 36849, USA; [b] Auburn University Pharmaceutical Care Center, Auburn University, 2155 Walker Building, Auburn, AL 36849, USA
* Corresponding author.
E-mail address: mcdowld@auburn.edu

Physician Assist Clin 8 (2023) 391–404
https://doi.org/10.1016/j.cpha.2022.10.015 physicianassistant.theclinics.com

patients in obtaining their medications. This article will provide a brief review of the medication-approval process, health and prescription drug insurance, and ways to assist patients with limited or no insurance.

FOOD AND DRUG ADMINISTRATION DRUG-APPROVAL PROCESS

The Food and Drug Administration (FDA) ensures that food supplies, cosmetics, and radiation-emitting products meet adequate safety standards for consumer use. Additionally, the agency certifies the safety, efficacy, and security of human and veterinary drugs, biological products, and medical devices.[6] Despite its primary role in the drug-approval process, the FDA does not develop, produce, or test drug products. Instead, drug manufacturers collect data from their sponsored research and clinical trials and submit it for FDA evaluation.[7]

Pharmaceuticals

New pharmaceutical products must undergo the FDA's 5-step drug-approval process, including brand name and generic prescription drugs, over-the-counter (OTC) products, human vaccines, and biologics. This structured approach allows the agency to ensure drugs are safe and effective before and after they are available to the public.[8,9] **Fig. 1** illustrates the FDA's 5-step drug-approval process and indicates where the Investigational new drug (IND) application, new drug application (NDA), and abbreviated new drug application (ANDA) are involved.

Herbal Supplements and Vitamins

Although the FDA regulates dietary supplements, they are considered food products and are not subject to the agency's drug-approval standards. Companies developing herbal supplements and vitamins may market and distribute these products without proving their safety or efficacy. However, once dietary supplements enter the marketplace, manufacturers are responsible for submitting mandatory adverse effect reports to the FDA. The FDA monitors its MedWatch program, which receives voluntary reports of serious adverse effects by the public and health-care providers.[13] If a dietary supplement is adulterated, misbranded, or poses a substantial risk to consumers, the FDA is authorized to intervene on behalf of public safety. Unlawful marketing of dietary supplements as a treatment, prevention, or cure for a disease can also be challenged by the FDA, and the agency has the authority to review drug labels, package inserts, and associated text materials.[14] **Box 1** highlights the main difference between pharmaceutical and dietary supplement-approval processes.

Insurance

Currently, about 30 million Americans do not have health insurance.[16] Lack of health and prescription drug insurance can result in medication nonadherence and poor health outcomes. In 2010, the Affordable Care Act (ACA) was enacted to regulate health insurance costs with the goal of making health insurance more affordable and accessible to more people.[17] Health insurance offers people assistance in paying for medical care and services, such as hospital stays, preventive care services, and medications. Health insurance coverage and costs vary and include government-funded programs and privately funded programs.

Medicare

Medicare is a health insurance program that is funded by the federal government.[18] Three groups of people are eligible to qualify for Medicare:[18]

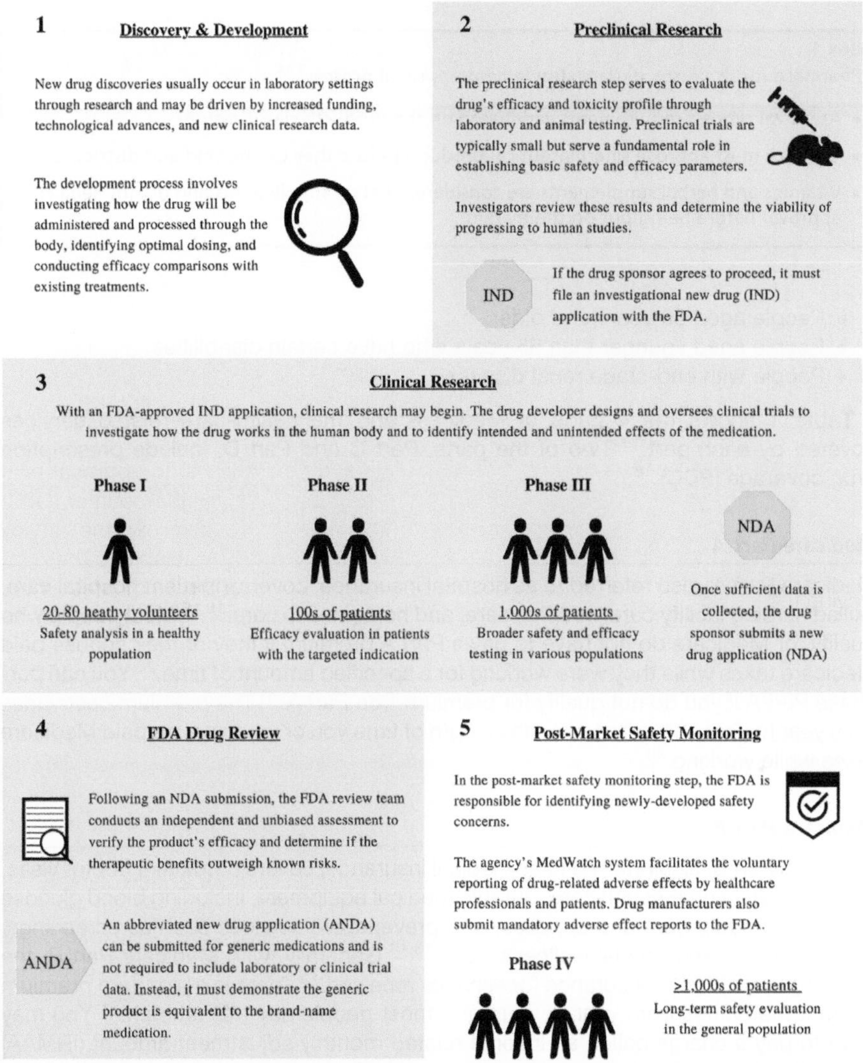
1
Discovery & Development
New drug discoveries usually occur in laboratory settings through research and may be driven by increased funding, technological advances, and new clinical research data.
The development process involves investigating how the drug will be administered and processed through the body, identifying optimal dosing, and conducting efficacy comparisons with existing treatments.
2
Preclinical Research
The preclinical research step serves to evaluate the drug's efficacy and toxicity profile through laboratory and animal testing. Preclinical trials are typically small but serve a fundamental role in establishing basic safety and efficacy parameters.
Investigators review these results and determine the viability of progressing to human studies.
IND
If the drug sponsor agrees to proceed, it must file an investigational new drug (IND) application with the FDA.
3
Clinical Research
With an FDA-approved IND application, clinical research may begin. The drug developer designs and oversees clinical trials to investigate how the drug works in the human body and to identify intended and unintended effects of the medication.
Phase I
20-80 heathy volunteers
Safety analysis in a healthy population
Phase II
100s of patients
Efficacy evaluation in patients with the targeted indication
Phase III
1,000s of patients
Broader safety and efficacy testing in various populations
NDA
Once sufficient data is collected, the drug sponsor submits a new drug application (NDA)
4
FDA Drug Review
Following an NDA submission, the FDA review team conducts an independent and unbiased assessment to verify the product's efficacy and determine if the therapeutic benefits outweigh known risks.
ANDA
An abbreviated new drug application (ANDA) can be submitted for generic medications and is not required to include laboratory or clinical trial data. Instead, it must demonstrate the generic product is equivalent to the brand-name medication.
5
Post-Market Safety Monitoring
In the post-market safety monitoring step, the FDA is responsible for identifying newly-developed safety concerns.
The agency's MedWatch system facilitates the voluntary reporting of drug-related adverse effects by healthcare professionals and patients. Drug manufacturers also submit mandatory adverse effect reports to the FDA.
Phase IV
≥1,000s of patients
Long-term safety evaluation in the general population

Fig. 1. FDA drug-approval process. The FDA's 5-step drug-approval process is a methodological operation that takes an average of 12 years. Drug manufacturers subsidize expenses involving discovery and development, animal studies, and human clinical research. Preceding clinical trials, drug sponsors must submit an IND application to the FDA. IND submissions seek FDA clearance to transport unapproved drugs to investigators and research sites across state lines. Moreover, IND submissions authorize human administration of an investigational drug.[10] Once drug manufacturers collect adequate safety and efficacy data substantiating their product, an NDA is submitted to the FDA. The NDA offers sufficient information for the FDA to evaluate the new product and assess if its benefits outweigh known risks. The agency must also review a package insert proposal to ensure accuracy, and manufacturing plans to certify the drug's quality, purity, and dose are upheld throughout its production.[11] Generic drug manufacturers can submit an ANDA requesting FDA approval to manufacture and market a generic drug. Because brand-name drug manufacturers completed the FDA's 5-step drug-approval process, generic drug manufacturers are exempt from developing clinical trial data, saving them time and money. Consequently, generic drugs are more affordable partly due to their abbreviated approval process.[12] ©igorkrasnoselskyi via Canva.com ©Icons8 via Canva.com ©Maxicons via Canva.com.

Box 1
Pharmaceuticals versus dietary supplement-approval process[7,15]

- Approval process requirements vary based on the product's classification
- The FDA must approve pharmaceutical products before they can be sold and distributed
- Vitamins and herbal supplements are considered dietary supplements and do not need FDA approval before being put on the market

- People aged 65 years and older
- People aged younger than 65 years who have certain disabilities
- People with end-stage renal disease

Table 1 shows the 4 parts of Medicare and the health-care–related services covered by each part.[18] Two of the parts, Part C and Part D, include prescription drug coverage (PDC).[18]

Medicare Part A

Medicare Part A, also referred to as hospital insurance, covers inpatient hospital care, skilled nursing facility care, hospice care, and home health care.[18,19] Most people who qualify for Medicare do not have to pay a Part A premium if they or their spouse paid Medicare taxes while they were working for a specified amount of time.[20] You can purchase Part A if you do not qualify for premium-free Part A.[20] The premium cost varies from year to year and is based on the length of time you or your spouse paid Medicare taxes while working.[20]

Medicare Part B

Medicare Part B, also referred to as medical insurance, covers outpatient doctor visits, medical tests, home health care, durable medical equipment, including blood glucose self-testing equipment and supplies, and preventative services such as screenings, immunizations, and annual wellness visits.[18,19] Generally, with Medicare Part B, the patient pays a 20% coinsurance for services received.[19] There is a standard premium amount that varies from year to year, and most people pay this amount.[21] You may have to pay a charge called an income related monthly adjustment amount (IRMAA) in addition to the standard premium if your modified adjusted gross income (MAGI) from your Internal Revenue Service tax return from 2 years ago is more than a certain threshold.[21]

Together, Medicare Parts A and B are referred to as "Original Medicare."[18] With Original Medicare, you may select to use any hospital and provider that accepts Medicare; therefore, you are not limited by a network of options.[19] If you have Original Medicare and would like to receive PDC, then you must join a Medicare Part D plan.[19]

Medicare Supplement Insurance

Medicare Supplement Insurance, also referred to as Medigap policies, are supplemental insurance policies sold by private insurance companies to help patients with Original Medicare cover costs, including copayments, coinsurance, and deductibles.[22] Patients pay an additional premium for their Medigap policy on top of their Part B premium.[22] Beginning in 2006, Medigap policies do not include PDC.[22]

Table 1
Medicare parts and covered services[18]

Medicare Part	Common Name	Covered Services
A	Hospital insurance	• Inpatient hospital care • Skilled nursing facility care • Hospice care • Some home health
B	Medical insurance	• Outpatient doctor visits • Medical tests • Home health care • Durable medical equipment • Screenings • Immunizations • Annual wellness visits
C	Medicare advantage plan	• Inpatient and outpatient care • Prescription drugs • Additional services (dental, vision, hearing, wellness)
D	PDC	• Prescription drugs • Immunizations

Medicare Part C

Medicare Part C is also referred to as Medicare Advantage Plans.[19] Although offered by private insurance companies, these plans must follow Medicare guidelines.[19] **Table 2** shows the 4 general types of Medicare Advantage Plans and if PDC is included.[19,22] If your income is above a certain amount, you will pay an IRMAA in addition to your premium.[23]

Medicare Part D

Medicare Part D, also referred to as drug coverage, is offered by private insurance companies.[19] Similar to Medicare Advantage Plans, Medicare Part D plans must follow Medicare guidelines.[19] With most plans, you will pay a monthly premium, which varies by plan, and you may pay an additional Part D IRMAA if your income is more than a set limit.[28] The 2022 average national monthly premium is approximately

Table 2
Medicare advantage plan types[23–27]

Plan Type	Prescription Drug Coverage
Health Maintenance Organization Plan	• Most plans include PDC • If you choose a plan without PDC, you cannot join a stand-alone Medicare Part D plan
Preferred Provider Organization Plan	• Most plans include PDC • If you choose a plan without PDC, you cannot join a stand-alone Medicare Part D plan
Private Fee-for-Service Plan	• Most plans include PDC • If you choose a plan without PDC, you can join a stand-alone Medicare Part D plan
Special Needs Plan (SNP)	• All SNPs offer PDC

US$33.[29] Deductibles also vary by plan, ranging from 0 to US$400.[29] Premiums, deductibles, and costs for medications can change from year to year. Plans send patients an Annual Notice of Change each fall to notify them of any changes for the following year.[29] Patients should consider all costs when selecting a drug plan. Patients may compare Medicare Part D and Medicare Advantage Plans by going to the website https://medicare.gov/plan-compare.

Another cost associated with Medicare Part D plans is a late enrollment penalty.[30] Patients may incur this penalty if they do not enroll in a plan during their initial enrollment period or if their PDC has lapsed for 63 or more consecutive days.[30] The penalty exits to encourage patients to enroll in Medicare Part D if they do not currently have credible PDC. The penalty amount depends on the length of time you have continued without credible PDC and is calculated by multiplying the number of months you do not have credible PDC by the national base beneficiary premium, which varies by year.[30] This amount is added to the cost of your monthly premium and legally considered part of the premium.[30] You will pay this penalty for as long as you are enrolled in a Medicare drug plan.

Patients who cannot afford their Medicare Part D plan costs, including premiums, deductibles, and coinsurance may qualify for Medicare Extra Help.[31] With Extra Help, patients either pay less or nothing at all for their premium and deductible.[31] Regarding copays and coinsurance, limits are set each year for generic drugs and brand-name drugs that are covered, and patients pay no more than those set amounts.[31] You may automatically qualify for Extra Help if you have Medicare and receive any of the following:[31]

- Medicaid coverage (full)
- Assistance from Medicaid paying your Medicare Part B premiums
- Supplemental Security Income benefits

In addition to those who automatically qualify for Extra Help, you may apply for Extra Help if you meet certain income and resource limits.[31]

Medicare Part D Coverage Gap

When patients enrolled in Medicare Part D plans reach a certain spending limit for covered drugs, they enter the coverage gap, commonly referred to as the "donut hole."[32] The spending limit can change from year to year.[32] Patients who receive Extra Help do not enter the coverage gap.[32] Once you enter the coverage gap, you will be responsible for paying no more than 25% of drug costs.[32] Once you spend a certain amount out of pocket, you exit the coverage gap. **Table 3** shows the costs that count toward the coverage gap versus those that do not.

Table 3
Costs counting toward coverage gap versus costs that do not count toward coverage gap[32]

Costs that Count Toward Coverage Gap	Costs that Do Not Count Toward Coverage Gap
• Deductible • Coinsurance • Copayments • Brand name drug discount received while in coverage gap • Amount you pay while in coverage gap	• Premium • Pharmacy dispensing fee • Amount you pay for drugs not covered by the plan

Once you pay a certain amount of eligible costs while in the coverage gap, you automatically move out of the coverage gap and into catastrophic coverage.[33] Once you reach catastrophic coverage, you will pay significantly lower coinsurance or copayment amounts for your prescription drugs for the remainder of the calendar year.[33] **Fig. 2** depicts the 4 Medicare Part D PDC phases and costs.

Medicaid

Medicaid is a health insurance program that is jointly funded by the federal and state government.[34] It is the largest health coverage program in the United States, providing coverage to more than 72 million Americans.[34] Populations eligible to qualify for Medicaid include the following:[34]

- Children
- Pregnant women
- Seniors
- Patients with disabilities
- Low-income patients

The ACA expanded the Medicaid program to cover more patients and established criteria for determining eligibility.[34] Eligibility for most patients is based on a patient's MAGI.[34] The Social Security Administration determines eligibility for patients who are aged 65 years and older, blind, or have a disability.[34]

Federal law stipulates that PDC is an optional benefit for patients but all states provide PDC for outpatient prescription drugs.[35] Each state has its own prescription drug formulary and sets copayment prices for medications.[36] For preferred drugs, the maximum allowable copayment is US$4.00 regardless of the federal poverty level (FPL).[36] The maximum allowable copayment for nonpreferred drugs depends on the FPL.[35] For patients with a family income of 100% to 150% FPL, the maximum

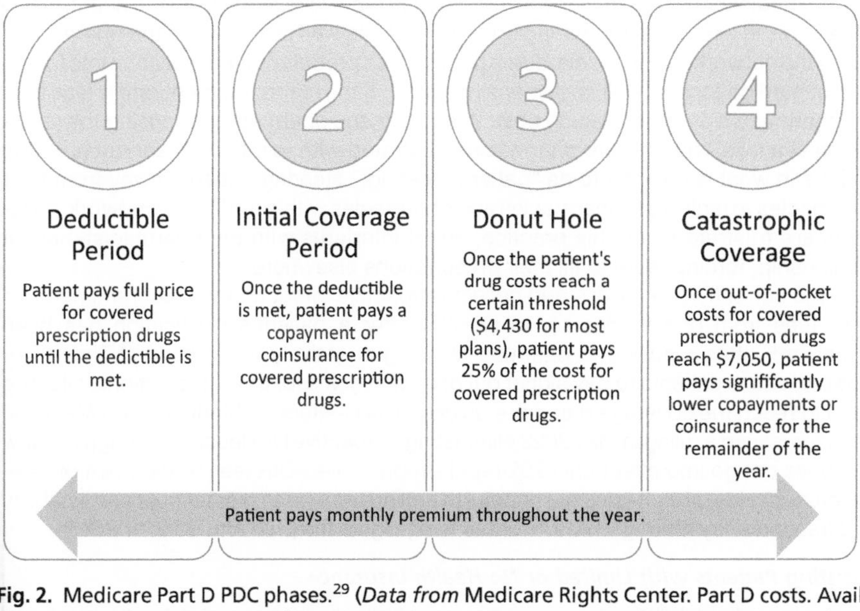

Fig. 2. Medicare Part D PDC phases.[29] (*Data from* Medicare Rights Center. Part D costs. Available at: https://www.medicareinteractive.org/get-answers/medicare-prescription-drug-coverage-partd/medicare-part-d-costs/part-d-costs. Accessed June 20, 2022.)

copayment is US$8.00, and it is 20% of the agency's cost if the family income is greater than 150%.[36]

Private Insurance

In addition to federal-funded and state-funded prescription drug programs, employers may also offer prescription drug insurance as a part of their employee benefits. Approximately 155 million people have employer-sponsored insurance.[37] Not all employer-sponsored health insurance plans cover prescription drugs.[38] With most employer-sponsored plans, the employer and the individual contribute to the insurance premium, and the individual pays a copayment for prescription drugs.[37]

Pharmacy Benefits Managers

Pharmacy benefits mangers (PBMs) are third-party administrators that act as intermediaries between drug manufacturers, health insurance companies, and pharmacies.[39] Beginning in the 1960s, the primary role of PBMs was processing prescription drug claims with the goal to reduce the cost of prescription drugs.[40] Since then, roles of PBMs have expanded to include other services, including mail-order pharmacy, selection of medications for prescription drug formularies, and adherence management.[40] PBMs create a network of pharmacies and offer pharmacies predetermined rates for reimbursement and dispensing fees.[41] Approximately 80% of patients in the United States receive benefits from a PBM.[41] These PBMs are the top 3 in the United States and account for approximately 78% of the present market:[41]

1. Caremark (CVS Health)
2. Express Scripts (Cigna)
3. OptumRx (United Health Group)

PBMs have come under scrutiny due to their lack of transparency in reporting their revenue. PBMs negotiate with drug manufacturers and receive rebates in exchange for adding medications to formularies.[39] PBMs also receive revenue from the health insurance plans in exchange for managing drug costs as well as fees from the pharmacies within the network.[39] PBMs reimburse pharmacies predetermined, set amounts for the cost of medications as well as dispensing fees.[41] If the reimbursement rate is less than the pharmacy's drug acquisition cost, it results in the pharmacy dispensing the medication at a loss. Not only are pharmacies frustrated with reimbursement rates, PBMs engage in what is referred to as "patient steering," steering patients away from their pharmacies to mail order pharmacies and pharmacies within the PBM's network.[42] Patients are frustrated with this practice, and it interferes with the pharmacist–patient relationship, forcing them to fill their prescriptions elsewhere.

PBMs currently can assess and collect retroactive direct and indirect remuneration (DIR) fees from pharmacies up to months after a patient's medication has been dispensed, often resulting in pharmacies being negatively reimbursed.[43] These DIR fees can cause patients to pay higher out of pocket costs for their medications, allowing them to reach the coverage gap more quickly. The Centers for Medicare and Medicaid Services issued a ruling in May 2022 eliminating retroactive DIR fees.[43] Although the new rule does not go into effect until 2024 and simply moves DIR fees to the point of sale-negotiated price, pharmacies are hopeful the ruling will lead to greater cost predictability and transparency among PBMs.[43] **Table 4** highlights the pros and cons of PBMs.

Assisting Patients with Limited or No Health Insurance

Medication affordability is a concern for many individuals. According to a Kaiser Family Foundation poll from 2021, 26% of Americans reported having difficulties paying for

Table 4
Pros and cons of PBMs[39–43]

Pros	Cons
• Negotiate reduced dispensing fees among pharmacies within networks • Negotiate rebates with drug manufacturers to reduce drug prices	• Reimburse pharmacies below drug acquisition cost and the cost to dispense the prescription • Develop formularies of covered medications, influencing which medications patients use • Assess retroactive DIR fees on pharmacies up to months after prescriptions are filled • Steer patients to mail order pharmacies or pharmacies within the PBM's network

their prescriptions, and 83% of adults perceive prescription costs to be unreasonably high. Additionally, 29% of patients stated that they did not take their medications as prescribed within the previous year because of prescription costs, including cutting tablets in half, skipping doses, not filling their prescription, or seeking OTC alternatives.[44] Moreover, the US Census Bureau reported that 28 million Americans did not have health insurance in 2020.[45]

Social Determinants of Health and Medication Access

Even with insurance, prescription coverage depends on the patient's specific plan, the insurance company's formulary, and other factors. Social determinants of health, such as education, income, transportation, access to nutritious foods, language, and literacy skills, play a crucial role in health and quality of life. For example, students struggling in school due to social or economic circumstances are less likely to pursue higher level education and may not be considered for employment offering health benefits packages. Additionally, individuals lacking financial stability may face challenges when picking up their medications, such as choosing between copays and other expenses. Furthermore, patients facing barriers to care are less inclined to invest in health insurance and have fewer preventive screenings, leading to risk factors increasing health-care costs, morbidity, and mortality.[46]

ASSISTANCE FROM DRUG MANUFACTURERS

Patient Assistance Programs

Pharmaceutical companies finance patient assistance programs (PAPs) to expand medication accessibility. Eligibility requirements vary by sponsoring drug companies; for example, some programs are reserved for uninsured individuals earning less than the FPL, whereas others offer relief for insured patients with high out-of-pocket costs and higher income limits. Once a PAP application is approved, patients can access certain medications at little or no cost. Sponsoring companies decide which drugs are available through their PAPs and establish benefit limitations, which are subject to change. Drug companies usually supply the most current and accurate PAP information on their website, serving as a valuable tool to determine medication availability, patient eligibility, and application requirements.[47] **Table 5** highlights the pros and cons of PAPs.

Copay Cards

Drug manufacturers also finance copay cards; however, unlike PAPs, copay cards primarily target patients with commercial insurance coverage.[48] Copay cards reduce

Table 5
Pros and cons of patient assistance programs[47]

Pros	Cons
• Patients may get medications at little or no cost • Some programs are accessible to patients without insurance • Certain programs reduce out-of-pocket costs for insured patients	• Eligibility requirements vary widely between sponsoring drug manufacturer and may be difficult for patients and providers to navigate • Extensive PAP applications can be challenging and limit the number of completed submissions • Uncertain sustainability since drug companies may remove medications from their PAPs at any time

insured patients' out-of-pocket costs for expensive, brand-name medications. In some cases, brand name prescriptions are more affordable to patients than generic alternatives due to copay card savings, which benefit the drug manufacturer through brand loyalty promotion. Commercial insurance coverage is required for copay card use because claims are first submitted to the patient's primary insurance and then followed by the copay card's benefits. As such, uninsured patients or those with government-funded insurance plans (Medicare, Medicaid, Tricare) are excluded from copay card benefits.

SUMMARY

The United States has set goals to increase the proportion of people with health and prescription drug insurance and has enacted regulations to increase access to affordable health care. Health insurance is a way for people to receive assistance paying for their medical care and services, including prescription drugs. Not all health insurance plans include PDC. Health insurance coverage and costs vary by program and include government-funded programs, such as Medicare and Medicaid, and privately funded programs. Uninsured or underinsured patients are less likely to take their medications as prescribed, leading to worse health outcomes. The FDA's drug-approval process enables the agency to protect public safety from ineffective and harmful medications. Pharmaceutical products are within the FDA's jurisdiction from the start, whereas vitamins and dietary supplements do not require FDA approval before they are approved, distributed, and sold across the country.

CLINICS CARE POINTS

- The FDA's new drug-approval process can be intricate and lengthy but it is essential to ensure that drugs are safe and effective for public use.
- Depending on certain qualifications, patients can have options for health and drug insurance through government-funded programs and private insurance companies to receive assistance in paying for medical care and services.
- PBMs serve as intermediaries between drug manufacturers, health insurance companies, and pharmacies and have come under scrutiny due to their lack of transparency in reporting their revenue, especially the rebates they receive from drug manufacturers.
- Millions of Americans face difficulties affording their prescriptions, and health outcomes are directly affected by reduced medication adherence.

DISCLOSURE

The authors have nothing to disclose.

REFERENCES

1. Centers for Disease Control and Prevention. Therapeutic drug use. Available at: https://www.cdc.gov/nchs/fastats/drug-use-therapeutic.htm. Accessed June 20, 2022.
2. Neiman AB, Ruppar T, Ho M, et al. CDC grand rounds: improving medication adherence for chronic disease management — innovations and opportunities. Morb Mortal Wkly Rep 2017;66(45):1248–51.
3. Healthy People 2030. Increase the proportion of people with health insurance – AHS-01. Available at: access-and-quality/increase-proportion-people-health-insurance-ahs-01">https://health.gov/healthypeople/objectives-and-data/browse-objectives/health-care-access-and-quality/increase-proportion-people-health-insurance-ahs-01. Accessed June 20, 2022.
4. Healthy People 2030. Increase the proportion of people with prescription drug insurance – AHS-03. Available at: access-and-quality/increase-proportion-people-prescription-drug-insurance-ahs-03">https://health.gov/healthypeople/objectives-and-data/browse-objectives/health-care-access-and-quality/increase-proportion-people-prescription-drug-insurance-ahs-03. Accessed June 20, 2022.
5. Healthy People 2030. Reduce the proportion of people who can't get prescription medicines when they need them – AHS-06. Available at: access-and-quality/reduce-proportion-people-who-cant-get-prescription-medicines-when-they-need-them-ahs-06">https://health.gov/healthypeople/objectives-and-data/browse-objectives/health-care-access-and-quality/reduce-proportion-people-who-cant-get-prescription-medicines-when-they-need-them-ahs-06. Accessed June 20, 2022.
6. United States Food and Drug Administration. What we do. Available at: https://www.fda.gov/about-fda/what-we-do. Accessed June 20, 2022.
7. United States Food and Drug Administration. Information for consumers on using dietary supplements. Available at: https://www.fda.gov/food/dietary-supplements/information-consumers-using-dietary-supplements. Accessed June 20, 2022.
8. United States Food and Drug Administration. Learn about drug and device approvals. Available at: https://www.fda.gov/patients/learn-about-drug-and-device-approvals. Accessed June 20, 2022.
9. United States Food and Drug Administration. The drug development process. Available at: https://www.fda.gov/patients/learn-about-drug-and-device-approvals/drug-development-process. Accessed June 20, 2022.
10. United States Food and Drug Administration. Investigational new drug (IND) application. Available at: https://www.fda.gov/drugs/types-applications/investigational-new-drug-ind-application. Accessed June 20, 2022.
11. United States Food and Drug Administration. New drug application (NDA). Available at: https://www.fda.gov/drugs/types-applications/new-drug-application-nda. Accessed June 20, 2022.
12. United States Food and Drug Administration. Abbreviated new drug application. Available at: https://www.fda.gov/drugs/types-applications/abbreviated-new-drug-application-anda. Accessed June 20, 2022.
13. United States Food and Drug Administration. MedWatch: the FDA safety information and adverse event reporting program. Available at: https://www.fda.gov/

safety/medwatch-fda-safety-information-and-adverse-event-reporting-program. Accessed June 20, 2022.
14. United States Food and Drug Administration. FDA 101: dietary supplements. Available at: https://www.fda.gov/consumers/consumer-updates/fda-101-dietary-supplements. Accessed on June 20, 2022.
15. United States Food and Drug Administration. Frequently asked questions about CDER. Available at: https://www.fda.gov/about-fda/center-drug-evaluation-and-research-cder/frequently-asked-questions-about-cder#1. Accessed June 20, 2022.
16. Healthy People 2030. Health insurance. Available at: https://health.gov/healthypeople/objectives-and-data/browse-objectives/health-insurance. Accessed June 20, 2022.
17. United States Centers for Medicare and Medicaid Services. Affordable Care Act (ACA). Available at: https://www.healthcare.gov/glossary/affordable-care-act/. Accessed June 20, 2022.
18. United States Centers for Medicare and Medicaid Services. What's Medicare?. Available at: https://www.medicare.gov/what-medicare-covers/your-medicare-coverage-choices/whats-medicare. Accessed June 20, 2022.
19. United States Centers for Medicare and Medicaid Services. Parts of Medicare. Available at: https://www.medicare.gov/basics/get-started-with-medicare/medicare-basics/parts-of-medicare. Accessed June 20, 2022.
20. United States Centers for Medicare and Medicaid Services. Part A costs. Available at: https://www.medicare.gov/your-medicare-costs/part-a-costs. Accessed June 20, 2022.
21. United States Centers for Medicare and Medicaid Services. Part B costs. Available at: https://www.medicare.gov/your-medicare-costs/part-b-costs. Accessed June 20, 2022.
22. United States Centers for Medicare and Medicaid Services. What's Medicare Supplement Insurance (Medigap)?. Available at: https://www.medicare.gov/supplements-other-insurance/whats-medicare-supplement-insurance-medigap. Accessed June 20, 2022.
23. United States Centers for Medicare and Medicaid Services. Medicare Advantage Plans. Available at: https://www.medicare.gov/sign-up-change-plans/types-of-medicare-health-plans/medicare-advantage-plans. Accessed June 20, 2022.
24. United States Centers for Medicare and Medicaid Services. Health Maintenance Organization (HMO). Available at: https://www.medicare.gov/sign-up-change-plans/types-of-medicare-health-plans/medicare-advantage-plans/health-maintenance-organization-hmo. Accessed June 20, 2022.
25. United States Centers for Medicare and Medicaid Services. Preferred Provider Organization (PPO). Available at: https://www.medicare.gov/sign-up-change-plans/types-of-medicare-health-plans/preferred-provider-organization-ppo. Accessed June 20, 2022.
26. United States Centers for Medicare and Medicaid Services. Private Fee-for-Service (PFFS) Plans. Available at: https://www.medicare.gov/sign-up-change-plans/types-of-medicare-health-plans/private-fee-for-service-pffs-plans. Accessed June 20, 2022.
27. United States Centers for Medicare and Medicaid Services. Special Needs Plans (SNPs). Available at: https://www.medicare.gov/sign-up-change-plans/types-of-medicare-health-plans/special-needs-plans-snp. Accessed June 20, 2022.
28. United States Centers for Medicare and Medicaid Services. Monthly premium for drug plans. Available at: https://www.medicare.gov/drug-coverage-part-d/costs-

for-medicare-drug-coverage/monthly-premium-for-drug-plans. Accessed June 20, 2022.
29. Medicare Rights Center. Part D costs. Available at: https://www.medicareinteractive.org/get-answers/medicare-prescription-drug-coverage-part-d/medicare-part-d-costs/part-d-costs. Accessed June 20, 2022.
30. United States Centers for Medicare and Medicaid Services. Part D late enrollment penalty. Available at: https://www.medicare.gov/drug-coverage-part-d/costs-for-medicare-drug-coverage/part-d-late-enrollment-penalty. Accessed June 20, 2022.
31. United States Centers for Medicare and Medicaid Services. Lower prescription costs. Available at: https://www.medicare.gov/your-medicare-costs/get-help-paying-costs/lower-prescription-costs. Accessed June 20, 2022.
32. United States Centers for Medicare and Medicaid Services. Costs in the coverage gap. Available at: https://www.medicare.gov/drug-coverage-part-d/costs-for-medicare-drug-coverage/costs-in-the-coverage-gap. Accessed June 20, 2022.
33. United States Centers for Medicare and Medicaid Services. Catastrophic coverage. Available at: https://www.medicare.gov/drug-coverage-part-d/costs-for-medicare-drug-coverage/catastrophic-coverage. Accessed June 20, 2022.
34. United States Centers for Medicare and Medicaid Services. Eligibility. Available at: https://www.medicaid.gov/medicaid/eligibility/index.html. Accessed June 20, 2022.
35. United States Centers for Medicare and Medicaid Services. Prescription drugs. Available at: https://www.medicaid.gov/medicaid/prescription-drugs/index.html. Accessed June 20, 2022.
36. United States Centers for Medicare and Medicaid Services. Cost sharing out of pocket costs. Available at: https://www.medicaid.gov/medicaid/cost-sharing/cost-sharing-out-pocket-costs/index.html. Accessed June 20, 2022.
37. Kaiser Family Foundation. 2021 employer health benefits survey. Available at: https://www.kff.org/report-section/ehbs-2021-summary-of-findings/. Accessed June 20, 2022.
38. Humana. Understanding how pharmacy benefits work. Available at: https://www.humana.com/employer/group-benefits-101/how-to-choose-plans/understanding-how-pharmacy-benefits-work. Accessed June 20, 2022.
39. Health Affairs. Health policy brief: pharmacy benefit managers. 2017. doi:10.1377/hpb2017.13
40. Burns LR. Contracting for prescription drug benefits: role of employers, insurers, and pharmacy benefit managers. In: The U.S. Healthcare Ecosystem: Payers, Providers, Producers. New York: McGraw Hill; 2021.
41. Taddei-Allen P. Evolution of the pharmacy benefit manager/community pharmacy relationship: an opportunity for success. J Manag Care Spec Pharm 2020;26(6): 708–10. https://doi.org/10.18553/jmcp.2020.26.6.708.
42. National Community Pharmacists Association. Patient steering. Available at: https://ncpa.org/patient-steering. Accessed June 20, 2022.
43. American Pharmacists Association. CMS eliminates retroactive DIR fees. Available at: https://www.pharmacist.com/Advocacy/Issues/CMS-Eliminates-Retroactive-DIR-Fees#:~:text=CMS%20issued%20a%20final%20rule,pays%20at%20the%20pharmacy%20counter. Accessed June 20, 2022.
44. Hamel L, Lopes L, Kirzinger A, et al. Public opinion on prescription drugs and their prices. Kaiser Fam Found. Available at: https://www.kff.org/health-costs/

poll-finding/public-opinion-on-prescription-drugs-and-their-prices/. Accessed June 20, 2022.
45. Keisler-Starkey K, Bunch LN. Health insurance coverage in the United States: 2020. United States Census Bureau. Available at: https://www.census.gov/library/publications/2021/demo/p60-274.html. Accessed June 20, 2022.
46. Healthy People 2030. Social determinants of health. Available at: https://health.gov/healthypeople/objectives-and-data/social-determinants-health. Accessed June 20, 2022.
47. NeedyMeds. Prescription assistance. Available at: https://www.needymeds.org/pap. Accessed June 20, 2022.
48. NeedyMeds. Co-pay cards FAQs. Available at: https://www.needymeds.org/copay-cards-faqs. Accessed June 20, 2022.

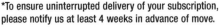

Printed and bound by CPI Group (UK) Ltd, Croydon, CR0 4YY
03/10/2024
01040847-0014